# *PARKINSON'S DISEASE DIET COOKBOOK FOR BEGINNERS 2024*

*Comprehensive Guide to Parkinson Brain Disorder Management for the Newly Diagnosed (Combining Recipes, Food Guides, Meal Plans, and Lifestyle Tips to Reverse Symptoms*

## Dr. Sarah Matthews

1

## A Heartfelt Note of Gratitude

Dear Reader,

Thank you from the bottom of my heart for choosing to embark on this journey through the **Parkinson's Disease Diet Cookbook for Beginners**. Your decision to learn more about Parkinson's disease and explore the role of nutrition in managing its symptoms is a testament to your dedication to health, well-being, and the pursuit of a better quality of life.

Whether you are a person living with Parkinson's, a caregiver, or someone seeking to support a loved one, your commitment to understanding and applying these dietary principles is truly commendable. This cookbook is designed to empower you with the knowledge, tools, and delicious recipes needed to make informed decisions that support your health journey.

I am deeply grateful for your time, interest, and effort in exploring the potential of nutrition to transform lives. Your willingness to educate yourself about Parkinson's disease and to embrace a holistic approach to managing its symptoms is a powerful step towards fostering resilience, vitality, and hope.

May this book serve as a valuable resource, inspiring you to create nourishing meals, cultivate healthy habits, and approach each day with optimism and confidence.

With heartfelt thanks,

Dr. Sarah Matthews.

# TABLE OF CONTENTS

# Introduction

## 1. Welcome to the Parkinson's Disease Diet Cookbook

### Understanding Parkinson's Disease

Parkinson's disease is a progressive neurodegenerative disorder that affects movement control. It is characterized by symptoms such as tremors, rigidity, bradykinesia (slowness of movement), and postural instability. The disease is caused by the gradual loss of dopamine-producing neurons in the brain, particularly in the substantia nigra region. Dopamine is a neurotransmitter that plays a crucial role in coordinating smooth and balanced muscle movements.

### The Importance of Diet and Nutrition

While there is no cure for Parkinson's disease, research has shown that diet and nutrition can play a significant role in managing symptoms and potentially slowing the progression of the disease. A well-balanced diet can help support overall brain health, improve motor function, and enhance quality of life for individuals with Parkinson's.

A diet rich in antioxidants, anti-inflammatory foods, and specific nutrients can help protect neurons, reduce oxidative stress, and support dopamine production. Additionally, proper nutrition can help manage non-motor symptoms such as constipation, mood changes, and sleep disturbances, which are common in Parkinson's patients.

## How to Use This Book

This cookbook is designed to be a comprehensive guide for individuals newly diagnosed with Parkinson's disease. It combines practical dietary advice, delicious recipes, and lifestyle tips to help manage symptoms and improve overall well-being.

Each section of the book is structured to provide you with the knowledge and tools you need to make informed dietary choices. You'll find:

- **Detailed Nutritional Guidelines:** Learn about the key nutrients that support brain health and how to incorporate them into your diet.
- **Easy-to-Follow Recipes:** Enjoy a variety of recipes that are not only nutritious but also simple to prepare, catering to different dietary preferences and restrictions.
- **Meal Planning and Preparation Tips:** Get practical advice on how to plan and prepare meals that fit your lifestyle and meet your nutritional needs.
- **Lifestyle Strategies:** Discover ways to enhance your overall health through exercise, stress management, and other wellness practices.

Whether you are cooking for yourself or for a loved one with Parkinson's, this book will empower you to take control of your diet and support your journey towards better health.

# PART I



## 2. What is Parkinson's Disease?

# Overview of Parkinson's Disease

Parkinson's disease (PD) is a chronic and progressive neurodegenerative disorder primarily affecting movement control. It results from the loss of dopamine-producing neurons in a part of the brain called the substantia nigra. Dopamine is a neurotransmitter essential for transmitting signals within the brain to produce smooth, purposeful movements. As PD progresses, the dopamine levels continue to drop, leading to more pronounced symptoms.

The exact cause of Parkinson's disease is still unknown, but it is believed to be a combination of genetic and environmental factors. Mutations in specific genes such as LRRK2, PARK7, PINK1, PRKN, and SNCA have been linked to PD. Environmental exposures such as pesticides, heavy metals, and head trauma are also associated with an increased risk of developing the disease.

# Symptoms and Diagnosis

**Motor Symptoms:**

- **Tremor:** One of the most recognizable symptoms, often starting in a hand or finger. This resting tremor can spread to other parts of the body and typically worsens with stress or anxiety.

- **Bradykinesia:** Slowness of movement that makes everyday tasks difficult and time-consuming. This symptom can lead to a reduction in spontaneous movements and a characteristic shuffling gait.
- **Rigidity:** Stiffness and inflexibility of the limbs and trunk. This can be accompanied by muscle pain and can reduce the range of motion.
- **Postural Instability:** Problems with balance and coordination, which increase the risk of falls. This symptom often appears in the later stages of the disease.

**Non-Motor Symptoms:**

- **Cognitive Changes:** Difficulty with memory, problem-solving, and attention. Some patients may develop Parkinson's disease dementia.
- **Mood Disorders:** Depression, anxiety, and apathy are common and can significantly impact quality of life.
- **Sleep Disturbances:** Insomnia, REM sleep behavior disorder (acting out dreams), and excessive daytime sleepiness.
- **Autonomic Dysfunction:** Problems with blood pressure regulation, bladder and bowel control, and sexual dysfunction.
- **Sensory Symptoms:** Loss of sense of smell, pain, and fatigue.

**Diagnosis:** There is no definitive test for Parkinson's disease, making diagnosis challenging. It is primarily based on medical history and a neurological examination. Criteria for diagnosis include the presence of two or more cardinal motor symptoms (tremor, bradykinesia, rigidity, postural instability) and a positive response to dopaminergic medications. Imaging tests such as DaTscan (dopamine transporter scan) can support the diagnosis by showing reduced dopamine activity in the brain.

# Stages of Parkinson's Disease

Parkinson's disease progresses through five stages, known as the Hoehn and Yahr scale:

1.  **Stage One:**
    o   Symptoms are mild and typically affect only one side of the body.
    o   Minimal or no functional impairment.
    o   Slight tremor, stiffness, or slowness of movement.
2.  **Stage Two:**
    o   Symptoms affect both sides of the body.
    o   No balance impairment, but daily activities may become more difficult.
    o   Increased rigidity and bradykinesia.
3.  **Stage Three:**
    o   Balance impairment becomes more pronounced.
    o   Increased risk of falls.
    o   Symptoms significantly affect daily activities, but patients remain independent.
4.  **Stage Four:**
    o   Severe disability.
    o   Patients may still walk or stand without assistance, but movement is greatly impaired.
    o   Assistance with daily activities is often needed.
5.  **Stage Five:**
    o   The most advanced stage.
    o   Patients are typically unable to stand or walk.

- o Require full-time assistance for all activities of daily living.
- o May experience severe cognitive impairments and hallucinations.

## 3. The Role of Diet in Parkinson's Management

# How Diet Affects Brain Health

Diet plays a crucial role in managing Parkinson's disease and supporting overall brain health. Nutrients from food can influence brain function, protect against oxidative stress, and help manage symptoms. A balanced diet can provide the necessary vitamins, minerals, and antioxidants to support neuronal health and dopamine production.

**Key Dietary Components:**

- **Antioxidants:** Combat oxidative stress, which is elevated in Parkinson's disease. Foods rich in antioxidants include berries, nuts, dark leafy greens, and other colorful fruits and vegetables.
- **Omega-3 Fatty Acids:** These essential fats have anti-inflammatory properties and support brain health. Sources include fatty fish (like salmon, mackerel, and sardines), flaxseeds, chia seeds, and walnuts.
- **Fiber:** Helps manage constipation, a common non-motor symptom of Parkinson's. High-fiber foods include whole grains, fruits, vegetables, and legumes.
- **Flavonoids:** Plant compounds that have been shown to have neuroprotective effects. Found in foods such as berries, citrus fruits, onions, and dark chocolate.

12

- **Vitamin D:** Important for bone health and may have a role in brain function. Sources include fortified foods, fatty fish, and exposure to sunlight.
- **Vitamin E:** An antioxidant that may help protect neurons. Found in nuts, seeds, and green leafy vegetables.
- **Coenzyme Q10:** An antioxidant that may improve mitochondrial function. Found in meat, fish, and whole grains.

# Nutrients That Support Neurological Function

**Protein and Amino Acids:**

- **Tyrosine:** An amino acid that is a precursor to dopamine. Found in high-protein foods like chicken, turkey, fish, dairy products, nuts, and seeds.
- **Phenylalanine:** Another amino acid that converts to tyrosine and ultimately to dopamine. Found in soy products, meat, fish, dairy, nuts, and seeds.

**B Vitamins:**

- **Vitamin B6:** Essential for dopamine synthesis. Found in foods such as chickpeas, potatoes, bananas, and fortified cereals.
- **Vitamin B12:** Important for neurological function and preventing anemia. Found in meat, fish, dairy, and fortified plant-based milks and cereals.
- **Folate (Vitamin B9):** Supports brain health and DNA synthesis. Found in leafy greens, legumes, nuts, and fortified grains.

**Minerals:**

- **Iron:** Necessary for dopamine synthesis. Found in red meat, beans, lentils, spinach, and fortified cereals.
- **Magnesium:** Supports muscle and nerve function. Found in nuts, seeds, whole grains, and green leafy vegetables.
- **Zinc:** Supports immune function and may have neuroprotective effects. Found in meat, shellfish, legumes, and seeds.

**Hydration:**

- Adequate water intake is crucial for overall health and helps manage symptoms such as constipation and low blood pressure. Aim for at least 8 cups of water a day, and more if active or in a hot climate.

# Foods to Avoid

While certain foods and nutrients can support brain health and manage symptoms, other foods may exacerbate symptoms or interact negatively with medications.

**Foods to Limit or Avoid:**

- **Processed Foods:** Often high in unhealthy fats, sugar, and sodium, which can contribute to inflammation and other health issues.
- **Saturated Fats and Trans Fats:** Found in fried foods, baked goods, and many processed snacks. These fats can increase inflammation and may worsen symptoms.
- **Excessive Protein:** Can interfere with the absorption of levodopa, a common medication used to treat Parkinson's

symptoms. Balance protein intake throughout the day rather than consuming large amounts at once.

- **High-Sugar Foods:** Can lead to rapid spikes and drops in blood sugar levels, which can affect energy levels and mood.
- **Caffeine:** While moderate caffeine intake may be beneficial for some, excessive amounts can interfere with sleep and exacerbate anxiety.

# PART II

*GETTING STARTED WITH THE PARKINSON'S DIET*

## 4. Essential Nutritional Guidelines

## Balanced Diet Principles

A balanced diet for individuals with Parkinson's disease includes a variety of foods from all food groups to ensure adequate nutrient intake. Here are the key principles to follow:

1. **Fruits and Vegetables:**
   - Aim for at least 5 servings of fruits and vegetables daily. These provide essential vitamins, minerals, fiber, and antioxidants.
   - Include a variety of colors to ensure a range of nutrients.
2. **Whole Grains:**
   - Choose whole grains over refined grains to increase fiber intake and support digestive health.
   - Examples include whole wheat, brown rice, quinoa, oats, and barley.
3. **Lean Proteins:**
   - Incorporate lean protein sources such as poultry, fish, beans, lentils, tofu, and low-fat dairy.
   - Balance protein intake throughout the day to avoid interference with levodopa absorption.
4. **Healthy Fats:**
   - Include sources of healthy fats such as olive oil, avocados, nuts, and seeds.

      o  Limit intake of saturated and trans fats.

5. **Dairy or Alternatives:**
   - o  Include low-fat dairy products or fortified plant-based alternatives for calcium and vitamin D.

6. **Hydration:**
   - o  Drink plenty of water throughout the day to stay hydrated and support bodily functions.

# Key Nutrients for Parkinson's Patients

**Antioxidants:** Combat oxidative stress, which can damage brain cells.

- Sources: Berries, nuts, dark leafy greens, colorful fruits, and vegetables.

**Omega-3 Fatty Acids:** Support brain health and reduce inflammation.

- Sources: Fatty fish (salmon, mackerel), flaxseeds, chia seeds, walnuts.

**Fiber:** Helps manage constipation.

- Sources: Whole grains, fruits, vegetables, legumes.

**Flavonoids:** Plant compounds with neuroprotective effects.

- Sources: Berries, citrus fruits, onions, dark chocolate.

**Vitamin D:** Important for bone health and may support brain function.

- Sources: Fortified foods, fatty fish, sunlight exposure.

**Vitamin E:** An antioxidant that may protect neurons.

- Sources: Nuts, seeds, green leafy vegetables.

**Coenzyme Q10:** May improve mitochondrial function.

- Sources: Meat, fish, whole grains.

**Tyrosine:** Precursor to dopamine.

- Sources: Chicken, turkey, fish, dairy, nuts, seeds.

**Phenylalanine:** Converts to tyrosine.

- Sources: Soy products, meat, fish, dairy, nuts, seeds.

**Vitamin B6:** Essential for dopamine synthesis.

- Sources: Chickpeas, potatoes, bananas, fortified cereals.

**Vitamin B12:** Important for neurological function.

- Sources: Meat, fish, dairy, fortified plant-based milks, cereals.

**Folate:** Supports brain health.

- Sources: Leafy greens, legumes, nuts, fortified grains.

**Iron:** Necessary for dopamine synthesis.

- Sources: Red meat, beans, lentils, spinach, fortified cereals.

18

**Magnesium:** Supports muscle and nerve function.

- Sources: Nuts, seeds, whole grains, green leafy vegetables.

**Zinc:** Supports immune function and may have neuroprotective effects.

- Sources: Meat, shellfish, legumes, seeds.

**Hydration:** Important for overall health.

- Aim for at least 8 cups of water a day, more if active or in a hot climate.

## 5. Pantry Essentials

# Must-Have Ingredients

Stocking your pantry with nutritious and versatile ingredients is key to maintaining a healthy diet for managing Parkinson's disease. Here are essential items to keep on hand:

**Whole Grains:**

- Brown rice, quinoa, oats, barley, whole wheat pasta, and whole grain bread.

**Lean Proteins:**

- Chicken, turkey, fish, eggs, tofu, tempeh, beans, lentils, and low-fat dairy.

**Healthy Fats:**

- Olive oil, avocado oil, coconut oil, nuts, seeds, and nut butters.

**Fruits and Vegetables:**

- Fresh, frozen, and dried fruits and vegetables. Include a variety of colors for a range of nutrients.

**Herbs and Spices:**

- Garlic, ginger, turmeric, cinnamon, oregano, basil, and other herbs and spices to add flavor and health benefits.

**Dairy or Alternatives:**

- Low-fat milk, yogurt, cheese, or fortified plant-based alternatives like almond milk, soy milk, and coconut yogurt.

**Other Essentials:**

- Canned tomatoes, vegetable broth, whole grain crackers, and high-fiber cereals.

# Shopping Tips for a Parkinson's-Friendly Diet

- **Plan Ahead:** Create a shopping list based on your weekly meal plan to avoid impulse purchases and ensure you have all the necessary ingredients.
- **Choose Whole Foods:** Opt for fresh, whole foods over processed and packaged items.

20

- **Read Labels:** Check for added sugars, unhealthy fats, and sodium levels in packaged foods.
- **Buy in Bulk:** Purchase staples like grains, beans, nuts, and seeds in bulk to save money and reduce packaging waste.
- **Seasonal and Local:** Buy seasonal and locally grown produce for better taste, nutrition, and sustainability.

# Reading Food Labels

Understanding food labels can help you make healthier choices. Look for:

- **Serving Size:** Be mindful of the serving size and how many servings are in a package.
- **Calories:** Consider the calories per serving and how it fits into your daily calorie needs.
- **Nutrients:** Check for key nutrients like fiber, protein, vitamins, and minerals.
- **Ingredients List:** Choose products with a short list of recognizable ingredients. Avoid items with added sugars, artificial additives, and trans fats.

## 6. Meal Planning and Preparation

# Creating a Weekly Meal Plan

A well-thought-out meal plan can help you maintain a balanced diet, save time and money, and reduce stress around meal times. Here's how to create a Parkinson's-friendly meal plan:

1. **Set Goals:** Determine your nutritional needs and goals, taking into account any dietary restrictions or preferences.

2. **Plan Meals:** Designate specific meals for each day of the week, considering variety and balance. Include a mix of protein, carbohydrates, healthy fats, fruits, and vegetables.
3. **Make a Shopping List:** Based on your meal plan, create a detailed shopping list of all the ingredients you'll need for the week.
4. **Prep Ingredients:** Wash, chop, and portion out ingredients in advance to streamline cooking during the week.
5. **Batch Cooking:** Cook large batches of staple foods like grains, beans, and proteins that can be used in multiple meals throughout the week.
6. **Flexibility:** Be flexible with your meal plan and adjust as needed based on changes in schedule, appetite, or ingredient availability.
7. **Plan for Leftovers:** Cook extra servings to have leftovers for future meals or lunches.
8. **Variety:** Include a variety of flavors, textures, and cuisines to keep meals interesting and enjoyable.

## Weekly Meal Plans

Creating weekly meal plans is an effective way to ensure you're consuming a balanced diet that supports the management of Parkinson's disease. These plans are designed to provide essential nutrients, and make meal preparation straightforward and enjoyable. Below are detailed weekly meal plans, each consisting of breakfasts, lunches, dinners, and snacks.

# Week 1

## Day 1

- **Breakfast:** Berry Blast Smoothie
    - *Ingredients:* 1 cup mixed berries, 1 banana, 1 cup almond milk, 1 tablespoon chia seeds, 1 tablespoon honey
    - *Instructions:* Blend all ingredients until smooth. Serve immediately.
- **Lunch:** Quinoa Salad with Chickpeas and Avocado
    - *Ingredients:* 1 cup cooked quinoa, 1 can chickpeas (drained and rinsed), 1 avocado (diced), 1 cup cherry tomatoes (halved), 1/4 cup red onion (diced), 2 tablespoons olive oil, juice of 1 lemon, salt and pepper to taste
    - *Instructions:* Combine all ingredients in a large bowl and toss gently. Serve chilled.
- **Dinner:** Salmon with Quinoa and Roasted Vegetables
    - *Ingredients:* 4 salmon fillets, 1 cup cooked quinoa, 2 cups mixed vegetables (such as bell peppers, zucchini, and carrots), 2 tablespoons olive oil, 1 teaspoon dried thyme, salt and pepper to taste
    - *Instructions:* Preheat oven to 400°F (200°C). Toss vegetables with olive oil, thyme, salt, and pepper. Spread on a baking sheet and roast for 20-25 minutes. Cook salmon fillets in a skillet over medium heat for 4-5 minutes per side. Serve salmon with quinoa and roasted vegetables.
- **Snack:** Apple Slices with Peanut Butter
    - *Ingredients:* 1 apple (sliced), 2 tablespoons peanut butter

- *Instructions:* Slice the apple and serve with peanut butter for dipping.

## Day 2

- **Breakfast:** Vegetable Omelette
    - *Ingredients:* 3 eggs, 1/4 cup diced bell peppers, 1/4 cup diced tomatoes, 1/4 cup spinach (chopped), salt and pepper to taste, 1 tablespoon olive oil
    - *Instructions:* Heat olive oil in a pan over medium heat. Sauté the vegetables until tender. Whisk the eggs with salt and pepper, pour into the pan, and cook until the eggs are set. Fold and serve.
- **Lunch:** Turkey and Veggie Wrap
    - *Ingredients:* 1 whole grain wrap, 4 slices turkey breast, 1/4 cup shredded lettuce, 1/4 cup sliced cucumber, 1/4 cup shredded carrots, 1 tablespoon hummus
    - *Instructions:* Spread hummus on the wrap, then layer with turkey, lettuce, cucumber, and carrots. Roll up and serve.
- **Dinner:** Eggplant and Chickpea Curry
    - *Ingredients:* 1 eggplant (diced), 1 can chickpeas (drained and rinsed), 1 onion (diced), 2 cloves garlic (minced), 1 tablespoon curry powder, 1 teaspoon cumin, 1 teaspoon coriander, 1/2 teaspoon turmeric, 1/4 teaspoon cayenne pepper, 1 can diced tomatoes, 1 cup vegetable broth, salt and pepper to taste, 2 tablespoons olive oil
    - *Instructions:* Heat olive oil in a large skillet over medium heat. Add eggplant and cook until softened. Add onion and garlic; cook until onion is translucent. Stir in spices and cook until fragrant. Add tomatoes,

chickpeas, and broth. Simmer for 20 minutes. Serve with rice.

- **Snack:** Greek Yogurt with Berries and Granola
  - *Ingredients:* 1 cup Greek yogurt, 1/2 cup mixed berries, 1/4 cup granola, 1 tablespoon honey
  - *Instructions:* Layer yogurt, berries, and granola in a bowl. Drizzle with honey and serve.

## Day 3

- **Breakfast:** Overnight Oats
  - *Ingredients:* 1/2 cup rolled oats, 1/2 cup almond milk, 1/4 cup Greek yogurt, 1 tablespoon chia seeds, 1 tablespoon honey, 1/2 cup mixed berries
  - *Instructions:* Combine all ingredients in a jar, cover, and refrigerate overnight. Serve chilled.
- **Lunch:** Lentil Soup
  - *Ingredients:* 1 cup lentils, 1 onion (diced), 2 carrots (diced), 2 celery stalks (diced), 3 cloves garlic (minced), 1 can diced tomatoes, 6 cups vegetable broth, 1 teaspoon cumin, 1 teaspoon paprika, salt and pepper to taste, 2 tablespoons olive oil
  - *Instructions:* Heat olive oil in a large pot over medium heat. Sauté onion, carrots, and celery until tender. Add garlic and cook until fragrant. Stir in lentils, tomatoes, and broth. Season with cumin, paprika, salt, and pepper. Bring to a boil, then simmer for 30-40 minutes until lentils are tender.
- **Dinner:** Lemon Herb Chicken with Brown Rice
  - *Ingredients:* 4 chicken breasts, 1/4 cup olive oil, 2 tablespoons lemon juice, 2 cloves garlic (minced), 1 teaspoon dried oregano, 1 teaspoon dried thyme, salt

and pepper to taste, 2 cups cooked brown rice, steamed vegetables

- o *Instructions:* Marinate chicken in olive oil, lemon juice, garlic, oregano, thyme, salt, and pepper for at least 30 minutes. Preheat oven to 375°F (190°C). Bake chicken for 25 minutes. Serve with brown rice and steamed vegetables.

- **Snack:** Carrot Sticks with Hummus
  - o *Ingredients:* 4 large carrots (peeled and cut into sticks), 1 cup hummus
  - o *Instructions:* Serve carrot sticks with hummus for dipping.

**Day 4**

- **Breakfast:** Greek Yogurt Parfait
  - o *Ingredients:* 1 cup Greek yogurt, 1/2 cup mixed berries, 1/4 cup granola, 1 tablespoon honey
  - o *Instructions:* Layer yogurt, berries, and granola in a bowl. Drizzle with honey and serve.
- **Lunch:** Spinach and Feta Stuffed Peppers
  - o *Ingredients:* 4 bell peppers (halved and seeded), 2 cups cooked quinoa, 1 cup spinach (chopped), 1/2 cup feta cheese (crumbled), 1/4 cup pine nuts, 2 tablespoons olive oil, salt and pepper to taste
  - o *Instructions:* Preheat oven to 375°F (190°C). Mix quinoa, spinach, feta, pine nuts, olive oil, salt, and pepper in a bowl. Stuff bell pepper halves with the mixture. Bake for 25-30 minutes until peppers are tender.
- **Dinner:** Vegetable Stir-Fry with Tofu
  - o *Ingredients:* 1 block firm tofu (drained and cubed), 2 tablespoons soy sauce, 1 tablespoon sesame oil, 2

cloves garlic (minced), 1 inch ginger (grated), 1 red bell pepper (sliced), 1 yellow bell pepper (sliced), 1 cup broccoli florets, 1 carrot (thinly sliced), 1/4 cup vegetable broth, 2 tablespoons hoisin sauce, cooked brown rice

- o *Instructions:* Marinate tofu in soy sauce for 10 minutes. Heat sesame oil in a skillet over medium-high heat. Cook tofu until golden. Remove and set aside. Add garlic and ginger to the skillet; sauté until fragrant. Add vegetables; stir-fry for 5-7 minutes. Return tofu to skillet, add broth and hoisin sauce. Cook for 2-3 minutes. Serve over brown rice.

- **Snack:** Trail Mix
  - o *Ingredients:* 1/2 cup almonds, 1/2 cup walnuts, 1/4 cup pumpkin seeds, 1/4 cup dried cranberries, 1/4 cup dark chocolate chips
  - o *Instructions:* Mix all ingredients in a bowl. Store in an airtight container. Enjoy a handful as a snack.

# Day 5

- **Breakfast:** Whole Grain Toast with Nut Butter
  - o *Ingredients:* 2 slices whole grain bread, 2 tablespoons almond or peanut butter
  - o *Instructions:* Toast bread and spread with nut butter. Serve immediately.
- **Lunch:** Chicken and Avocado Salad
  - o *Ingredients:* 2 cups mixed greens, 1 grilled chicken breast (sliced), 1 avocado (sliced), 1/2 cup cherry tomatoes (halved), 1/4 cup red onion (sliced), 2 tablespoons olive oil, juice of 1 lemon, salt and pepper to taste

- o *Instructions:* Combine all ingredients in a bowl and toss gently. Serve immediately.
- **Dinner:** Black Bean and Sweet Potato Tacos
  - o *Ingredients:* 2 large sweet potatoes (peeled and cubed), 1 can black beans (drained and rinsed), 1 red onion (diced), 1 teaspoon ground cumin, 1 teaspoon chili powder, salt and pepper to taste, corn or flour tortillas, optional toppings: avocado, salsa, cilantro, lime wedges
  - o *Instructions:* Preheat oven to 400°F (200°C). Toss sweet potato cubes with olive oil, cumin, chili powder, salt, and pepper. Spread on a baking sheet and roast for 25-30 minutes. Sauté onion until softened. Add black beans and cook until heated through. Warm tortillas and assemble tacos with sweet potatoes and black beans. Add optional toppings.
- **Snack:** Avocado Toast

  - *Ingredients:* 2 slices whole grain bread, 1 ripe avocado, salt and pepper to taste, optional: red pepper flakes, lemon juice, sliced tomatoes, poached egg
  - o *Instructions:* Toast the whole grain bread slices until golden brown. Mash the avocado in a bowl and season with salt and pepper. Spread the mashed avocado evenly on the toasted bread. Add any optional toppings such as red pepper flakes, a squeeze of lemon juice, sliced tomatoes, or a poached egg. Serve immediately.

**Day 6**

- **Breakfast:** Berry Blast Smoothie
  - *Ingredients:* 1 cup mixed berries, 1 banana, 1 cup almond milk, 1 tablespoon chia seeds, 1 tablespoon honey
  - *Instructions:* Blend all ingredients until smooth. Serve immediately.
- **Lunch:** Quinoa Salad with Chickpeas and Avocado
  - *Ingredients:* 1 cup cooked quinoa, 1 can chickpeas (drained and rinsed), 1 avocado (diced), 1 cup cherry tomatoes (halved), 1/4 cup red onion (diced), 2 tablespoons olive oil, juice of 1 lemon, salt and pepper to taste
  - *Instructions:* Combine all ingredients in a large bowl and toss gently. Serve chilled.
- **Dinner:** Salmon with Quinoa and Roasted Vegetables
  - *Ingredients:* 4 salmon fillets, 1 cup cooked quinoa, 2 cups mixed vegetables (such as bell peppers, zucchini, and carrots), 2 tablespoons olive oil, 1 teaspoon dried thyme, salt and pepper to taste
  - *Instructions:* Preheat oven to 400°F (200°C). Toss vegetables with olive oil, thyme, salt, and pepper. Spread on a baking sheet and roast for 20-25 minutes. Cook salmon fillets in a skillet over medium heat for 4-5 minutes per side. Serve salmon with quinoa and roasted vegetables.
- **Snack:** Apple Slices with Peanut Butter
  - *Ingredients:* 1 apple (sliced), 2 tablespoons peanut butter
  - *Instructions:* Slice the apple and serve with peanut butter for dipping.

**Day 7**

- **Breakfast:** Vegetable Omelette
  - *Ingredients:* 3 eggs, 1/4 cup diced bell peppers, 1/4 cup diced tomatoes, 1/4 cup spinach (chopped), salt and pepper to taste, 1 tablespoon olive oil
  - *Instructions:* Heat olive oil in a pan over medium heat. Sauté the vegetables until tender. Whisk the eggs with salt and pepper, pour into the pan, and cook until the eggs are set. Fold and serve.
- **Lunch:** Turkey and Veggie Wrap
  - *Ingredients:* 1 whole grain wrap, 4 slices turkey breast, 1/4 cup shredded lettuce, 1/4 cup sliced cucumber, 1/4 cup shredded carrots, 1 tablespoon hummus
  - *Instructions:* Spread hummus on the wrap, then layer with turkey, lettuce, cucumber, and carrots. Roll up and serve.
- **Dinner:** Eggplant and Chickpea Curry
  - *Ingredients:* 1 eggplant (diced), 1 can chickpeas (drained and rinsed), 1 onion (diced), 2 cloves garlic (minced), 1 tablespoon curry powder, 1 teaspoon cumin, 1 teaspoon coriander, 1/2 teaspoon turmeric, 1/4 teaspoon cayenne pepper, 1 can diced tomatoes, 1 cup vegetable broth, salt and pepper to taste, 2 tablespoons olive oil
  - *Instructions:* Heat olive oil in a large skillet over medium heat. Add eggplant and cook until softened. Add onion and garlic; cook until onion is translucent. Stir in spices and cook until fragrant. Add tomatoes, chickpeas, and broth. Simmer for 20 minutes. Serve with rice.

- **Snack:** Greek Yogurt with Berries and Granola
    - *Ingredients:* 1 cup Greek yogurt, 1/2 cup mixed berries, 1/4 cup granola, 1 tablespoon honey
    - *Instructions:* Layer yogurt, berries, and granola in a bowl. Drizzle with honey and serve.

# Week 2

## Day 1

- **Breakfast:** Overnight Oats
    - *Ingredients:* 1/2 cup rolled oats, 1/2 cup almond milk, 1/4 cup Greek yogurt, 1 tablespoon chia seeds, 1 tablespoon honey, 1/2 cup mixed berries
    - *Instructions:* Combine all ingredients in a jar, cover, and refrigerate overnight. Serve chilled.
- **Lunch:** Lentil Soup
    - *Ingredients:* 1 cup lentils, 1 onion (diced), 2 carrots (diced), 2 celery stalks (diced), 3 cloves garlic (minced), 1 can diced tomatoes, 6 cups vegetable broth, 1 teaspoon cumin, 1 teaspoon paprika, salt and pepper to taste, 2 tablespoons olive oil
    - *Instructions:* Heat olive oil in a large pot over medium heat. Sauté onion, carrots, and celery until tender. Add garlic and cook until fragrant. Stir in lentils, tomatoes, and broth. Season with cumin, paprika, salt, and pepper. Bring to a boil, then simmer for 30-40 minutes until lentils are tender.
- **Dinner:** Lemon Herb Chicken with Brown Rice
    - *Ingredients:* 4 chicken breasts, 1/4 cup olive oil, 2 tablespoons lemon juice, 2 cloves garlic (minced), 1 teaspoon dried oregano, 1 teaspoon dried thyme, salt

and pepper to taste, 2 cups cooked brown rice, steamed vegetables
  - *Instructions:* Marinate chicken in olive oil, lemon juice, garlic, oregano, thyme, salt, and pepper for at least 30 minutes. Preheat oven to 375°F (190°C). Bake chicken for 25 minutes. Serve with brown rice and steamed vegetables.
- **Snack:** Carrot Sticks with Hummus
  - *Ingredients:* 4 large carrots (peeled and cut into sticks), 1 cup hummus
  - *Instructions:* Serve carrot sticks with hummus for dipping.

## Day 2

- **Breakfast:** Greek Yogurt Parfait
  - *Ingredients:* 1 cup Greek yogurt, 1/2 cup mixed berries, 1/4 cup granola, 1 tablespoon honey
  - *Instructions:* Layer yogurt, berries, and granola in a bowl. Drizzle with honey and serve.
- **Lunch:** Spinach and Feta Stuffed Peppers
  - *Ingredients:* 4 bell peppers (halved and seeded), 2 cups cooked quinoa, 1 cup spinach (chopped), 1/2 cup feta cheese (crumbled), 1/4 cup pine nuts, 2 tablespoons olive oil, salt and pepper to taste
  - *Instructions:* Preheat oven to 375°F (190°C). Mix quinoa, spinach, feta, pine nuts, olive oil, salt, and pepper in a bowl. Stuff bell pepper halves with the mixture. Bake for 25-30 minutes until peppers are tender.
- **Dinner:** Vegetable Stir-Fry with Tofu
  - *Ingredients:* 1 block firm tofu (drained and cubed), 2 tablespoons soy sauce, 1 tablespoon sesame oil, 2

cloves garlic (minced), 1 inch ginger (grated), 1 red bell pepper (sliced), 1 yellow bell pepper (sliced), 1 cup broccoli florets, 1 carrot (thinly sliced), 1/4 cup vegetable broth, 2 tablespoons hoisin sauce, cooked brown rice

- o *Instructions:* Marinate tofu in soy sauce for 10 minutes. Heat sesame oil in a skillet over medium-high heat. Cook tofu until golden. Remove and set aside. Add garlic and ginger to the skillet; sauté until fragrant. Add vegetables; stir-fry for 5-7 minutes. Return tofu to skillet, add broth and hoisin sauce. Cook for 2-3 minutes. Serve over brown rice.

- **Snack:** Trail Mix
  - o *Ingredients:* 1/2 cup almonds, 1/2 cup walnuts, 1/4 cup pumpkin seeds, 1/4 cup dried cranberries, 1/4 cup dark chocolate chips
  - o *Instructions:* Mix all ingredients in a bowl. Store in an airtight container. Enjoy a handful as a snack.

## Day 3

- **Breakfast:** Whole Grain Toast with Nut Butter
  - o *Ingredients:* 2 slices whole grain bread, 2 tablespoons almond or peanut butter
  - o *Instructions:* Toast bread and spread with nut butter. Serve immediately.
- **Lunch:** Chicken and Avocado Salad
  - o *Ingredients:* 2 cups mixed greens, 1 grilled chicken breast (sliced), 1 avocado (sliced), 1/2 cup cherry tomatoes (halved), 1/4 cup red onion (sliced), 2 tablespoons olive oil, juice of 1 lemon, salt and pepper to taste

- o *Instructions:* Combine all ingredients in a bowl and toss gently. Serve immediately.
- **Dinner:** Black Bean and Sweet Potato Tacos
  - o *Ingredients:* 2 large sweet potatoes (peeled and cubed), 1 can black beans (drained and rinsed), 1 red onion (diced), 1 teaspoon ground cumin, 1 teaspoon chili powder, salt and pepper to taste, corn or flour tortillas, optional toppings: avocado, salsa, cilantro, lime wedges

*Instructions:* Preheat oven to 400°F (200°C). Toss sweet potato cubes with olive oil, cumin, chili powder, salt, and pepper. Spread on a baking sheet and roast on a baking sheet and roast for 25-30 minutes. Sauté onion until softened. Add black beans and cook until heated through. Warm tortillas and assemble tacos with sweet potatoes and black beans. Add optional toppings.

- **Snack:** Avocado Toast
  - o *Ingredients:* 2 slices whole grain bread, 1 ripe avocado, salt and pepper to taste, optional: red pepper flakes, lemon juice, sliced tomatoes, poached egg
  - o *Instructions:* Toast the whole grain bread slices until golden brown. Mash the avocado in a bowl and season with salt and pepper. Spread the mashed avocado evenly on the toasted bread. Add any optional toppings such as red pepper flakes, a squeeze of lemon juice, sliced tomatoes, or a poached egg. Serve immediately.

## Day 4

- **Breakfast:** Berry Blast Smoothie
  - *Ingredients:* 1 cup mixed berries, 1 banana, 1 cup almond milk, 1 tablespoon chia seeds, 1 tablespoon honey
  - *Instructions:* Blend all ingredients until smooth. Serve immediately.
- **Lunch:** Quinoa Salad with Chickpeas and Avocado
  - *Ingredients:* 1 cup cooked quinoa, 1 can chickpeas (drained and rinsed), 1 avocado (diced), 1 cup cherry tomatoes (halved), 1/4 cup red onion (diced), 2 tablespoons olive oil, juice of 1 lemon, salt and pepper to taste
  - *Instructions:* Combine all ingredients in a large bowl and toss gently. Serve chilled.
- **Dinner:** Salmon with Quinoa and Roasted Vegetables
  - *Ingredients:* 4 salmon fillets, 1 cup cooked quinoa, 2 cups mixed vegetables (such as bell peppers, zucchini, and carrots), 2 tablespoons olive oil, 1 teaspoon dried thyme, salt and pepper to taste
  - *Instructions:* Preheat oven to 400°F (200°C). Toss vegetables with olive oil, thyme, salt, and pepper. Spread on a baking sheet and roast for 20-25 minutes. Cook salmon fillets in a skillet over medium heat for 4-5 minutes per side. Serve salmon with quinoa and roasted vegetables.
- **Snack:** Apple Slices with Peanut Butter
  - *Ingredients:* 1 apple (sliced), 2 tablespoons peanut butter
  - *Instructions:* Slice the apple and serve with peanut butter for dipping.

## Day 5

- **Breakfast:** Vegetable Omelette
  - *Ingredients:* 3 eggs, 1/4 cup diced bell peppers, 1/4 cup diced tomatoes, 1/4 cup spinach (chopped), salt and pepper to taste, 1 tablespoon olive oil
  - *Instructions:* Heat olive oil in a pan over medium heat. Sauté the vegetables until tender. Whisk the eggs with salt and pepper, pour into the pan, and cook until the eggs are set. Fold and serve.
- **Lunch:** Turkey and Veggie Wrap
  - *Ingredients:* 1 whole grain wrap, 4 slices turkey breast, 1/4 cup shredded lettuce, 1/4 cup sliced cucumber, 1/4 cup shredded carrots, 1 tablespoon hummus
  - *Instructions:* Spread hummus on the wrap, then layer with turkey, lettuce, cucumber, and carrots. Roll up and serve.
- **Dinner:** Eggplant and Chickpea Curry
  - *Ingredients:* 1 eggplant (diced), 1 can chickpeas (drained and rinsed), 1 onion (diced), 2 cloves garlic (minced), 1 tablespoon curry powder, 1 teaspoon cumin, 1 teaspoon coriander, 1/2 teaspoon turmeric, 1/4 teaspoon cayenne pepper, 1 can diced tomatoes, 1 cup vegetable broth, salt and pepper to taste, 2 tablespoons olive oil
  - *Instructions:* Heat olive oil in a large skillet over medium heat. Add eggplant and cook until softened. Add onion and garlic; cook until onion is translucent. Stir in spices and cook until fragrant. Add tomatoes, chickpeas, and broth. Simmer for 20 minutes. Serve with rice.

- **Snack:** Greek Yogurt with Berries and Granola
  - *Ingredients:* 1 cup Greek yogurt, 1/2 cup mixed berries, 1/4 cup granola, 1 tablespoon honey
  - *Instructions:* Layer yogurt, berries, and granola in a bowl. Drizzle with honey and serve.

## Day 6

- **Breakfast:** Overnight Oats
  - *Ingredients:* 1/2 cup rolled oats, 1/2 cup almond milk, 1/4 cup Greek yogurt, 1 tablespoon chia seeds, 1 tablespoon honey, 1/2 cup mixed berries
  - *Instructions:* Combine all ingredients in a jar, cover, and refrigerate overnight. Serve chilled.
- **Lunch:** Lentil Soup
  - *Ingredients:* 1 cup lentils, 1 onion (diced), 2 carrots (diced), 2 celery stalks (diced), 3 cloves garlic (minced), 1 can diced tomatoes, 6 cups vegetable broth, 1 teaspoon cumin, 1 teaspoon paprika, salt and pepper to taste, 2 tablespoons olive oil
  - *Instructions:* Heat olive oil in a large pot over medium heat. Sauté onion, carrots, and celery until tender. Add garlic and cook until fragrant. Stir in lentils, tomatoes, and broth. Season with cumin, paprika, salt, and pepper. Bring to a boil, then simmer for 30-40 minutes until lentils are tender.
- **Dinner:** Lemon Herb Chicken with Brown Rice
  - *Ingredients:* 4 chicken breasts, 1/4 cup olive oil, 2 tablespoons lemon juice, 2 cloves garlic (minced), 1 teaspoon dried oregano, 1 teaspoon dried thyme, salt and pepper to taste, 2 cups cooked brown rice, steamed vegetables

- o *Instructions:* Marinate chicken in olive oil, lemon juice, garlic, oregano, thyme, salt, and pepper for at least 30 minutes. Preheat oven to 375°F (190°C). Bake chicken for 25 minutes. Serve with brown rice and steamed vegetables.
- **Snack:** Carrot Sticks with Hummus
  - o *Ingredients:* 4 large carrots (peeled and cut into sticks), 1 cup hummus
  - o *Instructions:* Serve carrot sticks with hummus for dipping.

## Day 7

- **Breakfast:** Greek Yogurt Parfait
  - o *Ingredients:* 1 cup Greek yogurt, 1/2 cup mixed berries, 1/4 cup granola, 1 tablespoon honey
  - o *Instructions:* Layer yogurt, berries, and granola in a bowl. Drizzle with honey and serve.
- **Lunch:** Spinach and Feta Stuffed Peppers
  - o *Ingredients:* 4 bell peppers (halved and seeded), 2 cups cooked quinoa, 1 cup spinach (chopped), 1/2 cup feta cheese (crumbled), 1/4 cup pine nuts, 2 tablespoons olive oil, salt and pepper to taste
  - o *Instructions:* Preheat oven to 375°F (190°C). Mix quinoa, spinach, feta, pine nuts, olive oil, salt, and pepper in a bowl. Stuff bell pepper halves with the mixture. Bake for 25-30 minutes until peppers are tender.
- **Dinner:** Vegetable Stir-Fry with Tofu
  - o *Ingredients:* 1 block firm tofu (drained and cubed), 2 tablespoons soy sauce, 1 tablespoon sesame oil, 2 cloves garlic (minced), 1 inch ginger (grated), 1 red bell pepper (sliced), 1 yellow bell pepper (sliced), 1

cup broccoli florets, 1 carrot (thinly sliced), 1/4 cup vegetable broth, 2 tablespoons hoisin sauce, cooked brown rice

- o *Instructions:* Marinate tofu in soy sauce for 10 minutes. Heat sesame oil in a skillet over medium-high heat. Cook tofu until golden. Remove and set aside. Add garlic and ginger to the skillet; sauté until fragrant. Add vegetables; stir-fry for 5-7 minutes. Return tofu to skillet, add broth and hoisin sauce. Cook for 2-3 minutes. Serve over brown rice.
- **Snack:** Trail Mix
  - o *Ingredients:* 1/2 cup almonds, 1/2 cup walnuts, 1/4 cup pumpkin seeds, 1/4 cup dried cranberries, 1/4 cup dark chocolate chips
  - o *Instructions:* Mix all ingredients in a bowl. Store in an airtight container. Enjoy a handful as a snack.

# Week 3

## Day 1

- **Breakfast:** Smoothie Bowl
  - o *Ingredients:* 1 cup frozen berries, 1 banana, 1/2 cup almond milk, 1 tablespoon chia seeds, 1 tablespoon honey, toppings: granola, sliced fruit, coconut flakes
  - o *Instructions:* Blend the frozen berries, banana, almond milk, chia seeds, and honey until smooth. Pour into a bowl and add toppings of choice. Serve immediately.
- **Lunch:** Mediterranean Chickpea Salad
  - o *Ingredients:* 1 can chickpeas (drained and rinsed), 1 cup cherry tomatoes (halved), 1 cucumber (diced), 1/4 cup red onion (diced), 1/4 cup kalamata olives

(sliced), 2 tablespoons olive oil, juice of 1 lemon, 1 teaspoon dried oregano, salt and pepper to taste

- o *Instructions:* Combine all ingredients in a large bowl and toss gently. Serve chilled.

- **Dinner:** Baked Cod with Asparagus and Quinoa
  - o *Ingredients:* 4 cod fillets, 1 bunch asparagus (trimmed), 2 tablespoons olive oil, 1 teaspoon garlic powder, 1 teaspoon lemon zest, salt and pepper to taste, 1 cup cooked quinoa
  - o *Instructions:* Preheat oven to 400°F (200°C). Arrange cod fillets and asparagus on a baking sheet. Drizzle with olive oil, and sprinkle with garlic powder, lemon zest, salt, and pepper. Bake for 15-20 minutes until fish flakes easily with a fork. Serve with cooked quinoa.
- **Snack:** Mixed Nuts and Seeds
  - o *Ingredients:* 1/4 cup almonds, 1/4 cup walnuts, 1/4 cup sunflower seeds, 1/4 cup pumpkin seeds
  - o *Instructions:* Mix all ingredients in a bowl. Store in an airtight container. Enjoy a handful as a snack.

## Day 2

- **Breakfast:** Banana Pancakes
  - o *Ingredients:* 1 banana (mashed), 2 eggs, 1/2 teaspoon baking powder, 1/4 teaspoon cinnamon, 1 teaspoon vanilla extract
  - o *Instructions:* Mix all ingredients until well combined. Heat a non-stick pan over medium heat and pour batter to form small pancakes. Cook until bubbles form on the surface, then flip and cook until golden

brown. Serve with fresh berries or a drizzle of maple syrup.

- **Lunch:** Tuna Salad Lettuce Wraps
  - *Ingredients:* 1 can tuna (drained), 1/4 cup Greek yogurt, 1 tablespoon Dijon mustard, 1/4 cup celery (diced), 1/4 cup red onion (diced), salt and pepper to taste, large lettuce leaves
  - *Instructions:* In a bowl, mix tuna, Greek yogurt, mustard, celery, and red onion. Season with salt and pepper. Spoon the tuna mixture onto large lettuce leaves and wrap. Serve immediately.
- **Dinner:** Turkey Meatballs with Spaghetti Squash
  - *Ingredients:* 1 spaghetti squash, 1 pound ground turkey, 1/4 cup breadcrumbs, 1/4 cup Parmesan cheese (grated), 1 egg, 2 cloves garlic (minced), 1 teaspoon Italian seasoning, salt and pepper to taste, 1 jar marinara sauce
  - *Instructions:* Preheat oven to 375°F (190°C). Cut spaghetti squash in half, remove seeds, and bake cut-side down on a baking sheet for 40 minutes. In a bowl, mix turkey, breadcrumbs, Parmesan, egg, garlic, Italian seasoning, salt, and pepper. Form into meatballs and bake on a separate baking sheet for 20 minutes. Warm marinara sauce in a pot, add baked meatballs, and simmer for 10 minutes. Use a fork to scrape spaghetti squash into strands and serve with meatballs and sauce.
- **Snack:** Veggie Sticks with Guacamole
  - *Ingredients:* 1 cucumber (sliced), 2 carrots (peeled and sliced), 1 red bell pepper (sliced), 1 cup guacamole

o *Instructions:* Arrange veggie sticks on a plate and serve with guacamole for dipping.

## Day 3

- **Breakfast:** Chia Pudding
  - o *Ingredients:* 1/4 cup chia seeds, 1 cup almond milk, 1 tablespoon maple syrup, 1/2 teaspoon vanilla extract, toppings: fresh berries, nuts
  - o *Instructions:* Combine chia seeds, almond milk, maple syrup, and vanilla extract in a bowl. Stir well and refrigerate overnight. Serve with toppings of choice.
- **Lunch:** Grilled Chicken and Veggie Skewers
  - o *Ingredients:* 2 chicken breasts (cubed), 1 red bell pepper (cubed), 1 yellow bell pepper (cubed), 1 red onion (cubed), 1 zucchini (sliced), 2 tablespoons olive oil, 1 teaspoon dried oregano, salt and pepper to taste
  - o *Instructions:* Preheat grill to medium-high heat. Thread chicken and vegetables onto skewers. Brush with olive oil and season with oregano, salt, and pepper. Grill for 10-15 minutes, turning occasionally, until chicken is cooked through and vegetables are tender.
- **Dinner:** Beef Stir-Fry with Broccoli and Brown Rice
  - o *Ingredients:* 1 pound beef sirloin (sliced thin), 2 cups broccoli florets, 1 red bell pepper (sliced), 2 cloves garlic (minced), 1 inch ginger (grated), 1/4 cup soy sauce, 2 tablespoons hoisin sauce, 1 tablespoon sesame oil, 1 cup cooked brown rice
  - o *Instructions:* Heat sesame oil in a large skillet over medium-high heat. Add beef and cook until browned. Remove and set aside. Add garlic, ginger, broccoli,

and bell pepper to the skillet; cook until vegetables are tender. Return beef to skillet, add soy sauce and hoisin sauce, and stir-fry for another 2-3 minutes. Serve over brown rice.

- **Snack:** Cottage Cheese with Pineapple
    - *Ingredients:* 1 cup cottage cheese, 1/2 cup pineapple chunks (fresh or canned)
    - *Instructions:* Combine cottage cheese and pineapple chunks in a bowl. Serve immediately.

## Day 4

- **Breakfast:** Spinach and Mushroom Frittata
    - *Ingredients:* 6 eggs, 1/4 cup milk, 1 cup spinach (chopped), 1/2 cup mushrooms (sliced), 1/4 cup feta cheese (crumbled), salt and pepper to taste, 1 tablespoon olive oil
    - *Instructions:* Preheat oven to 375°F (190°C). In an ovenproof skillet, heat olive oil over medium heat. Sauté spinach and mushrooms until tender. In a bowl, whisk eggs, milk, salt, and pepper. Pour over vegetables in the skillet and cook until edges are set. Sprinkle with feta and transfer to the oven. Bake for 10-15 minutes until the center is set. Serve warm.
- **Lunch:** Quinoa and Black Bean Stuffed Peppers
    - *Ingredients:* 4 bell peppers (halved and seeded), 1 cup cooked quinoa, 1 can black beans (drained and rinsed), 1/2 cup corn kernels, 1/4 cup red onion (diced), 1/4 cup cilantro (chopped), 2 tablespoons lime juice, salt and pepper to taste
    - *Instructions:* Preheat oven to 375°F (190°C). Mix quinoa, black beans, corn, onion, cilantro, lime juice, salt, and pepper in a bowl. Stuff bell pepper halves

with the mixture. Bake for 25-30 minutes until peppers are tender.

- **Dinner:** Shrimp and Vegetable Skewers with Couscous
  - *Ingredients:* 1 pound shrimp (peeled and deveined), 1 zucchini (sliced), 1 red bell pepper (cubed), 1 yellow bell pepper (cubed), 1 red onion (cubed), 2 tablespoons olive oil, 1 teaspoon smoked paprika, salt and pepper to taste, 1 cup cooked couscous
  - *Instructions:* Preheat grill to medium-high heat. Thread shrimp and vegetables onto skewers. Brush with olive oil and season with smoked paprika, salt, and pepper. Grill for 8-10 minutes, turning occasionally, until shrimp are opaque and vegetables are tender. Serve with cooked couscous.
- **Snack:** Apple Slices with Almond Butter
  - *Ingredients:* 1 apple (sliced), 2 tablespoons almond butter
  - *Instructions:* Slice the apple and serve with almond butter for dipping.

## Day 5

- **Breakfast:** Blueberry Muffins
  - *Ingredients:* 1 1/2 cups whole wheat flour, 1/2 cup rolled oats, 1/2 cup honey, 1/2 teaspoon baking soda, 1 teaspoon baking powder, 1/2 teaspoon salt, 1/2 teaspoon cinnamon, 1 cup Greek yogurt, 1/4 cup milk, 1/4 cup olive oil, 2 eggs, 1 teaspoon vanilla extract, 1 cup fresh blueberries
  - *Instructions:* Preheat oven to 375°F (190°C). In a bowl, combine flour, oats, baking soda, baking powder, salt, and cinnamon. In another bowl, mix yogurt, milk, olive oil, eggs, honey, and vanilla

extract. Combine wet and dry ingredients, fold in blueberries, and divide batter into a muffin tin. Bake for 20-25 minutes until golden brown.

- **Lunch:** Caprese Salad with Balsamic Glaze
  - *Ingredients:* 2 cups mixed greens, 2 tomatoes (sliced), 8 ounces fresh mozzarella (sliced), 1/4 cup fresh basil leaves, 2 tablespoons olive oil, 1 tablespoon balsamic glaze, salt and pepper to taste
  - *Instructions:* Arrange mixed greens on a plate. Top with tomato slices, mozzarella, and basil leaves. Drizzle with olive oil and balsamic glaze. Season with salt and pepper. Serve immediately.
- **Dinner:** Beef and Broccoli Stir-Fry
  - *Ingredients:* 1 pound beef sirloin (sliced thin), 2 cups broccoli florets, 1 red bell pepper (sliced), 2 cloves garlic (minced), 1 inch ginger (grated), 1/4 cup soy sauce, 2 tablespoons hoisin sauce, 1 tablespoon sesame oil, 1 cup cooked brown rice
  - *Instructions:* Heat sesame oil in a large skillet over medium-high heat. Add beef and cook until browned.

Remove beef and set aside. Add garlic, ginger, broccoli, and bell pepper to the skillet; cook until vegetables are tender. Return beef to skillet, add soy sauce and hoisin sauce, and stir-fry for another 2-3 minutes. Serve over cooked brown rice.

- **Snack:** Celery Sticks with Cream Cheese
  - *Ingredients:* 4 celery stalks (cut into sticks), 1/4 cup cream cheese
  - *Instructions:* Fill celery sticks with cream cheese. Serve immediately.

## Day 6

- **Breakfast:** Peanut Butter Banana Smoothie
  - *Ingredients:* 1 banana, 1 cup almond milk, 2 tablespoons peanut butter, 1 tablespoon chia seeds, 1 tablespoon honey
  - *Instructions:* Blend all ingredients until smooth. Serve immediately.
- **Lunch:** Greek Chicken Salad
  - *Ingredients:* 2 cups mixed greens, 1 cup cooked chicken breast (diced), 1/2 cup cherry tomatoes (halved), 1/2 cucumber (sliced), 1/4 cup red onion (sliced), 1/4 cup kalamata olives, 1/4 cup feta cheese (crumbled), 2 tablespoons olive oil, juice of 1 lemon, salt and pepper to taste
  - *Instructions:* Combine mixed greens, chicken, cherry tomatoes, cucumber, red onion, olives, and feta cheese in a bowl. Drizzle with olive oil and lemon juice. Season with salt and pepper. Toss gently and serve.
- **Dinner:** Baked Chicken with Brussels Sprouts and Sweet Potatoes
  - *Ingredients:* 4 chicken breasts, 1 pound Brussels sprouts (halved), 2 sweet potatoes (cubed), 2 tablespoons olive oil, 1 teaspoon garlic powder, 1 teaspoon paprika, salt and pepper to taste
  - *Instructions:* Preheat oven to 400°F (200°C). Arrange chicken, Brussels sprouts, and sweet potatoes on a baking sheet. Drizzle with olive oil, and season with garlic powder, paprika, salt, and pepper. Bake for 25-30 minutes until chicken is cooked through and vegetables are tender.

- **Snack:** Edamame with Sea Salt
  - *Ingredients:* 1 cup edamame (steamed), sea salt to taste
  - *Instructions:* Sprinkle sea salt over steamed edamame. Serve warm.

## Day 7

- **Breakfast:** Avocado and Tomato Toast
  - *Ingredients:* 2 slices whole grain bread, 1 ripe avocado, 1 tomato (sliced), salt and pepper to taste, 1 tablespoon olive oil
  - *Instructions:* Toast the bread slices until golden brown. Mash the avocado and season with salt and pepper. Spread avocado on toast, top with tomato slices, and drizzle with olive oil. Serve immediately.
- **Lunch:** Lentil and Vegetable Soup
  - *Ingredients:* 1 cup lentils, 1 onion (diced), 2 carrots (diced), 2 celery stalks (diced), 3 cloves garlic (minced), 1 can diced tomatoes, 6 cups vegetable broth, 1 teaspoon cumin, 1 teaspoon paprika, salt and pepper to taste, 2 tablespoons olive oil
  - *Instructions:* Heat olive oil in a large pot over medium heat. Sauté onion, carrots, and celery until tender. Add garlic and cook until fragrant. Stir in lentils, tomatoes, and broth. Season with cumin, paprika, salt, and pepper. Bring to a boil, then simmer for 30-40 minutes until lentils are tender.
- **Dinner:** Spaghetti with Marinara Sauce and Turkey Meatballs
  - *Ingredients:* 1 package whole grain spaghetti, 1 pound ground turkey, 1/4 cup breadcrumbs, 1/4 cup Parmesan cheese (grated), 1 egg, 2 cloves garlic

(minced), 1 teaspoon Italian seasoning, salt and pepper to taste, 1 jar marinara sauce

- o *Instructions:* Cook spaghetti according to package instructions. In a bowl, mix ground turkey, breadcrumbs, Parmesan, egg, garlic, Italian seasoning, salt, and pepper. Form into meatballs and bake at 375°F (190°C) for 20 minutes. Warm marinara sauce in a pot, add meatballs, and simmer for 10 minutes. Serve meatballs and sauce over cooked spaghetti.

- **Snack:** Fresh Fruit Salad
  - o *Ingredients:* 1 cup mixed fruit (such as berries, kiwi, mango, and pineapple), 1 tablespoon lime juice, 1 teaspoon honey
  - o *Instructions:* Combine mixed fruit in a bowl. Drizzle with lime juice and honey. Toss gently and serve.

# Week 4

**Day 1**

- **Breakfast:** Oatmeal with Berries and Nuts
  - o *Ingredients:* 1/2 cup rolled oats, 1 cup almond milk, 1/4 cup mixed berries, 1 tablespoon honey, 1/4 cup mixed nuts
  - o *Instructions:* Cook oats in almond milk according to package instructions. Top with berries, honey, and nuts. Serve immediately.

- **Lunch:** Hummus and Veggie Wrap
  - o *Ingredients:* 1 whole grain wrap, 1/4 cup hummus, 1/4 cup shredded lettuce, 1/4 cup sliced cucumber, 1/4 cup shredded carrots, 1/4 cup red bell pepper (sliced)

- o *Instructions:* Spread hummus on the wrap, then layer with lettuce, cucumber, carrots, and bell pepper. Roll up and serve.
- **Dinner:** Grilled Salmon with Quinoa and Steamed Vegetables
  - o *Ingredients:* 4 salmon fillets, 1 cup cooked quinoa, 2 cups mixed vegetables (such as broccoli, carrots, and snap peas), 2 tablespoons olive oil, 1 teaspoon garlic powder, salt and pepper to taste
  - o *Instructions:* Preheat grill to medium-high heat. Brush salmon with olive oil and season with garlic powder, salt, and pepper. Grill for 4-5 minutes per side. Serve with cooked quinoa and steamed vegetables.
- **Snack:** Greek Yogurt with Honey and Almonds
  - o *Ingredients:* 1 cup Greek yogurt, 1 tablespoon honey, 1/4 cup sliced almonds
  - o *Instructions:* Drizzle honey over Greek yogurt and sprinkle with sliced almonds. Serve immediately.

## Day 2

- **Breakfast:** Egg and Spinach Breakfast Burrito
  - o *Ingredients:* 1 whole grain tortilla, 2 eggs, 1/2 cup spinach (chopped), 1/4 cup shredded cheese, 1 tablespoon olive oil, salt and pepper to taste
  - o *Instructions:* Heat olive oil in a pan over medium heat. Scramble eggs with spinach until cooked. Season with salt and pepper. Place eggs and spinach in the tortilla, top with cheese, and roll up. Serve immediately.
- **Lunch:** Shrimp and Avocado Salad
  - o *Ingredients:* 2 cups mixed greens, 1 cup cooked shrimp, 1 avocado (diced), 1/4 cup cherry tomatoes

(halved), 2 tablespoons olive oil, juice of 1 lime, salt and pepper to taste

- o *Instructions:* Combine mixed greens, shrimp, avocado, and cherry tomatoes in a bowl. Drizzle with olive oil and lime juice. Season with salt and pepper. Toss gently and serve.

- **Dinner:** Turkey Chili
  - o *Ingredients:* 1 pound ground turkey, 1 onion (diced), 2 cloves garlic (minced), 1 bell pepper (diced), 1 can kidney beans (drained and rinsed), 1 can black beans (drained and rinsed), 1 can diced tomatoes, 2 tablespoons chili powder, 1 teaspoon cumin, 1 teaspoon paprika, salt and pepper to taste, 2 tablespoons olive oil
  - o *Instructions:* Heat olive oil in a large pot over medium heat. Cook onion, garlic, and bell pepper until tender. Add ground turkey and cook until browned. Stir in beans, tomatoes, chili powder, cumin, paprika, salt, and pepper. Simmer for 30 minutes. Serve warm.

- **Snack:** Cottage Cheese with Peaches
  - o *Ingredients:* 1 cup cottage cheese, 1/2 cup sliced peaches (fresh or canned)
  - o *Instructions:* Combine cottage cheese and sliced peaches in a bowl. Serve immediately.

## Day 3

- **Breakfast:** Smoothie Bowl
  - o *Ingredients:* 1 cup frozen berries, 1 banana, 1/2 cup almond milk, 1 tablespoon chia seeds, 1 tablespoon honey, toppings: granola, sliced fruit, coconut flakes

- o *Instructions:* Blend the frozen berries, banana, almond milk, chia seeds, and honey until smooth. Pour into a bowl and add toppings of choice. Serve immediately.
- **Lunch:** Grilled Chicken Caesar Salad
  - o *Ingredients:* 2 cups romaine lettuce (chopped), 1 grilled chicken breast (sliced), 1/4 cup Parmesan cheese (shaved), 1/4 cup croutons, 2 tablespoons Caesar dressing
  - o *Instructions:* Toss romaine lettuce with Caesar dressing. Top with sliced grilled chicken, Parmesan cheese, and croutons. Serve immediately.
- **Dinner:** Stuffed Bell Peppers with Quinoa and Ground Beef
  - o *Ingredients:* 4 bell peppers (halved and seeded), 1 cup cooked quinoa, 1/2 pound ground beef, 1/2 onion (diced), 1 cup diced tomatoes, 1/4 cup shredded cheese, 2 tablespoons olive oil, salt and pepper to taste

*Instructions:* Preheat oven to 375°F (190°C). In a skillet, heat olive oil over medium heat and cook ground beef with diced onion until browned. Stir in cooked quinoa and diced tomatoes. Season with salt and pepper. Stuff bell pepper halves with the mixture and place in a baking dish. Sprinkle with shredded cheese and bake for 25-30 minutes until peppers are tender and cheese is melted.

- **Snack:** Trail Mix
  - o *Ingredients:* 1/4 cup almonds, 1/4 cup dried cranberries, 1/4 cup cashews, 1/4 cup dark chocolate chips
  - o *Instructions:* Combine all ingredients in a bowl. Store in an airtight container and enjoy a handful as a snack.

**Day 4**

- **Breakfast:** Greek Yogurt Parfait
    - *Ingredients:* 1 cup Greek yogurt, 1/4 cup granola, 1/2 cup mixed berries, 1 tablespoon honey
    - *Instructions:* Layer Greek yogurt, granola, and mixed berries in a glass or bowl. Drizzle with honey and serve immediately.
- **Lunch:** Veggie and Hummus Sandwich
    - *Ingredients:* 2 slices whole grain bread, 1/4 cup hummus, 1/4 cup cucumber (sliced), 1/4 cup red bell pepper (sliced), 1/4 cup shredded carrots, 1/4 cup spinach leaves
    - *Instructions:* Spread hummus on both slices of bread. Layer cucumber, bell pepper, carrots, and spinach on one slice, then top with the other slice. Cut in half and serve.
- **Dinner:** Baked Tilapia with Lemon and Garlic
    - *Ingredients:* 4 tilapia fillets, 2 tablespoons olive oil, 2 cloves garlic (minced), juice of 1 lemon, salt and pepper to taste, 1/4 cup fresh parsley (chopped)
    - *Instructions:* Preheat oven to 375°F (190°C). Place tilapia fillets in a baking dish. Drizzle with olive oil, sprinkle with garlic, lemon juice, salt, and pepper. Bake for 20-25 minutes until fish is flaky. Garnish with fresh parsley and serve with a side of steamed vegetables or brown rice.
- **Snack:** Sliced Bell Peppers with Hummus
    - *Ingredients:* 1 red bell pepper (sliced), 1 yellow bell pepper (sliced), 1/4 cup hummus
    - *Instructions:* Serve bell pepper slices with hummus for dipping.

## Day 5

- **Breakfast:** Apple Cinnamon Overnight Oats
    - *Ingredients:* 1/2 cup rolled oats, 1/2 cup almond milk, 1/4 cup Greek yogurt, 1/2 apple (diced), 1/2 teaspoon cinnamon, 1 tablespoon honey
    - *Instructions:* Combine oats, almond milk, Greek yogurt, apple, cinnamon, and honey in a jar or bowl. Stir well, cover, and refrigerate overnight. Serve cold in the morning.
- **Lunch:** Quinoa Salad with Chickpeas and Feta
    - *Ingredients:* 1 cup cooked quinoa, 1 can chickpeas (drained and rinsed), 1/2 cucumber (diced), 1/2 red bell pepper (diced), 1/4 cup red onion (diced), 1/4 cup feta cheese (crumbled), 2 tablespoons olive oil, juice of 1 lemon, salt and pepper to taste
    - *Instructions:* In a large bowl, combine quinoa, chickpeas, cucumber, bell pepper, red onion, and feta cheese. Drizzle with olive oil and lemon juice, and season with salt and pepper. Toss gently and serve.
- **Dinner:** Chicken and Vegetable Stir-Fry
    - *Ingredients:* 2 chicken breasts (sliced thin), 2 cups mixed vegetables (such as broccoli, bell peppers, and snap peas), 2 cloves garlic (minced), 1 inch ginger (grated), 1/4 cup soy sauce, 1 tablespoon sesame oil, 1 tablespoon olive oil
    - *Instructions:* Heat olive oil in a large skillet over medium-high heat. Add chicken and cook until browned. Remove and set aside. In the same skillet, add sesame oil, garlic, and ginger; cook until fragrant. Add mixed vegetables and stir-fry until tender. Return chicken to the skillet and add soy sauce. Cook for

another 2-3 minutes until everything is heated through. Serve with brown rice or noodles.

- **Snack:** Hard-Boiled Eggs
  - *Ingredients:* 2 hard-boiled eggs
  - *Instructions:* Peel the eggs and enjoy as a protein-rich snack.

## Day 6

- **Breakfast:** Spinach and Feta Breakfast Wrap
  - *Ingredients:* 1 whole grain tortilla, 2 eggs, 1/2 cup spinach (chopped), 1/4 cup feta cheese (crumbled), 1 tablespoon olive oil, salt and pepper to taste
  - *Instructions:* Heat olive oil in a pan over medium heat. Scramble eggs with spinach until cooked. Season with salt and pepper. Place eggs and spinach in the tortilla, top with feta cheese, and roll up. Serve immediately.
- **Lunch:** Tuna Nicoise Salad
  - *Ingredients:* 2 cups mixed greens, 1 can tuna (drained), 1/4 cup green beans (blanched), 1/4 cup cherry tomatoes (halved), 1/4 cup olives, 1 hard-boiled egg (sliced), 2 tablespoons olive oil, juice of 1 lemon, salt and pepper to taste
  - *Instructions:* Arrange mixed greens on a plate. Top with tuna, green beans, cherry tomatoes, olives, and sliced egg. Drizzle with olive oil and lemon juice, and season with salt and pepper. Serve immediately.
- **Dinner:** Pork Tenderloin with Roasted Vegetables
  - *Ingredients:* 1 pork tenderloin, 2 cups mixed vegetables (such as carrots, potatoes, and Brussels sprouts), 2 tablespoons olive oil, 1 teaspoon garlic powder, 1 teaspoon rosemary, salt and pepper to taste

- *Instructions:* Preheat oven to 400°F (200°C). Place pork tenderloin and vegetables on a baking sheet. Drizzle with olive oil, and season with garlic powder, rosemary, salt, and pepper. Roast for 25-30 minutes until pork is cooked through and vegetables are tender. Let pork rest for a few minutes before slicing. Serve with the roasted vegetables.
- **Snack:** Mixed Berry Smoothie
  - *Ingredients:* 1 cup mixed berries, 1 banana, 1/2 cup Greek yogurt, 1/2 cup almond milk
  - *Instructions:* Blend all ingredients until smooth. Serve immediately.

## Day 7

- **Breakfast:** Avocado Toast with Poached Egg
  - *Ingredients:* 2 slices whole grain bread, 1 ripe avocado, 2 eggs, salt and pepper to taste, 1 tablespoon olive oil, 1 tablespoon white vinegar
  - *Instructions:* Toast the bread slices until golden brown. Mash the avocado and season with salt and pepper. Spread avocado on toast. To poach the eggs, bring a pot of water to a gentle simmer and add white vinegar. Crack eggs into the water and cook for 3-4 minutes until whites are set. Remove with a slotted spoon and place on avocado toast. Drizzle with olive oil and serve immediately.
- **Lunch:** Mediterranean Chickpea Salad
  - *Ingredients:* 1 can chickpeas (drained and rinsed), 1/2 cucumber (diced), 1/2 red bell pepper (diced), 1/4 cup red onion (diced), 1/4 cup kalamata olives (sliced), 1/4 cup feta cheese (crumbled), 2 tablespoons olive oil, juice of 1 lemon, salt and pepper to taste

- *Instructions:* In a large bowl, combine chickpeas, cucumber, bell pepper, red onion, olives, and feta cheese. Drizzle with olive oil and lemon juice, and season with salt and pepper. Toss gently and serve.
- **Dinner:** Baked Cod with Tomato and Basil
  - *Ingredients:* 4 cod fillets, 2 cups cherry tomatoes (halved), 1/4 cup fresh basil (chopped), 2 tablespoons olive oil, 2 cloves garlic (minced), salt and pepper to taste
  - *Instructions:* Preheat oven to 375°F (190°C). Place cod fillets in a baking dish. In a bowl, combine cherry tomatoes, basil, olive oil, and garlic. Season with salt and pepper. Spoon the tomato mixture over the cod fillets. Bake for 20-25 minutes until fish is flaky. Serve with a side of quinoa or brown rice.
- **Snack:** Roasted Chickpeas
  - *Ingredients:* 1 can chickpeas (drained and rinsed), 1 tablespoon olive oil, 1 teaspoon paprika, 1/2 teaspoon garlic powder, salt and pepper to taste
  - *Instructions:* Preheat oven to 400°F (200°C). Pat chickpeas dry with a paper towel. In a bowl, toss chickpeas with olive oil, paprika, garlic powder, salt, and pepper. Spread on a baking sheet and roast for 20-30 minutes until crispy. Let cool and enjoy as a snack.

## Tips for Simplifying Meal Prep

- **Use Convenience Foods:** Opt for pre-cut vegetables, canned beans, and frozen fruits for quick and easy meal prep.
- **Invest in Kitchen Tools:** Utilize kitchen gadgets like slow cookers, pressure cookers, and food processors to save time and effort.

- **Prep Ahead:** Take advantage of downtime to prep ingredients or cook meals in advance, such as on weekends or during less busy times of the day.
- **One-Pot Meals:** Choose recipes that can be made in a single pot or pan to minimize cleanup and simplify cooking.
- **Delegate Tasks:** Involve family members or caregivers in meal preparation to share the workload and make it a collaborative effort.

# Cooking Strategies for Ease and Convenience

- **Simple Recipes:** Choose recipes with minimal ingredients and straightforward instructions to make cooking more manageable.
- **Freezer-Friendly Meals:** Prepare large batches of meals and freeze individual portions for quick and convenient meals later on.
- **Meal Kits:** Consider using meal kit delivery services or pre-packaged meal solutions to save time on planning and shopping.
- **Healthy Swaps:** Make healthier substitutions in recipes, such as using Greek yogurt instead of sour cream or whole grain pasta instead of white pasta.

By following these meal planning and preparation strategies, you can simplify the process of cooking nutritious meals while managing Parkinson's disease.

# PART III

## *RECIPES*

## Nutritious Breakfast Options

Starting the day with a nutritious breakfast is essential for maintaining energy levels and supporting overall health. In this chapter, we'll explore a variety of breakfast options tailored to individuals managing Parkinson's disease.

1. **Green Power Smoothie**
   - *Ingredients:* 1 cup spinach, 1 banana, 1/2 cup pineapple chunks, 1/2 cup Greek yogurt, 1 tablespoon chia seeds, 1/2 cup almond milk.
   - *Instructions:* Blend all ingredients until smooth. Serve chilled.

2. **Berry Blast Smoothie**
   - *Ingredients:* 1/2 cup mixed berries (strawberries, blueberries, raspberries), 1/2 cup plain Greek yogurt, 1 tablespoon honey, 1/2 cup almond milk, 1 tablespoon flaxseeds.
   - *Instructions:* Blend all ingredients until smooth. Add ice if desired and blend again. Serve immediately.

3. **Tropical Paradise Smoothie**
   - *Ingredients:* 1/2 cup mango chunks, 1/2 cup pineapple chunks, 1/2 banana, 1/2 cup coconut milk, 1/4 cup orange juice, 1 tablespoon shredded coconut.
   - *Instructions:* Blend all ingredients until smooth. Garnish with shredded coconut before serving.

4. **Chocolate Peanut Butter Smoothie**
   - *Ingredients:* 1 tablespoon cocoa powder, 2 tablespoons peanut butter, 1 banana, 1/2 cup Greek yogurt, 1/2 cup almond milk, 1 tablespoon honey.
   - *Instructions:* Blend all ingredients until smooth. Add more milk if needed for desired consistency. Enjoy!
5. **Oatmeal Breakfast Smoothie**
   - *Ingredients:* 1/4 cup rolled oats, 1 banana, 1/2 cup mixed berries, 1/2 cup Greek yogurt, 1/2 cup almond milk, 1 tablespoon honey.
   - *Instructions:* Blend all ingredients until oats are fully incorporated and smooth. Serve immediately.

# High-Protein Breakfast Options

1. **Egg and Avocado Toast**
   - *Ingredients:* 2 slices whole grain bread, 2 eggs, 1 avocado, salt, and pepper to taste.
   - *Instructions:* Toast the bread slices. While toasting, fry or poach the eggs according to preference. Mash the avocado and spread it evenly on the toasted bread. Top with eggs and season with salt and pepper.
2. **Greek Yogurt Parfait**
   - *Ingredients:* 1 cup Greek yogurt, 1/4 cup granola, 1/2 cup mixed berries, 1 tablespoon honey.
   - *Instructions:* Layer Greek yogurt, granola, and mixed berries in a glass or bowl. Drizzle with honey and serve.
3. **Quinoa Breakfast Bowl**
   - *Ingredients:* 1/2 cup cooked quinoa, 1/4 cup Greek yogurt, 1/4 cup mixed nuts and seeds, 1/2 cup sliced

fruits (such as bananas, berries, or apples), honey or maple syrup for drizzling.

- *Instructions:* In a bowl, layer cooked quinoa, Greek yogurt, mixed nuts and seeds, and sliced fruits. Drizzle with honey or maple syrup before serving.

4. **Spinach and Feta Omelette**

- *Ingredients:* 2 eggs, 1 cup fresh spinach, 2 tablespoons crumbled feta cheese, salt, and pepper to taste.
- *Instructions:* Beat the eggs in a bowl and season with salt and pepper. Heat a non-stick skillet over medium heat and add the beaten eggs. Once the edges start to set, add spinach and feta cheese. Fold the omelette in half and cook until the eggs are fully set.

5. **Protein-Packed Pancakes**

- *Ingredients:* 1 cup oats, 1 banana, 1/2 cup Greek yogurt, 2 eggs, 1 teaspoon baking powder, 1/2 teaspoon cinnamon, toppings of choice (such as berries, nuts, or honey).
- *Instructions:* Blend oats, banana, Greek yogurt, eggs, baking powder, and cinnamon until smooth. Heat a non-stick pan over medium heat and pour batter to form pancakes. Cook until bubbles form on the surface, then flip and cook the other side. Serve with your favorite toppings.

# Easy-to-Prepare Breakfast Ideas

1. **Overnight Chia Seed Pudding**

- *Ingredients:* 1/4 cup chia seeds, 1 cup almond milk, 1 tablespoon honey, toppings of choice (such as sliced fruits or nuts).

- o *Instructions:* Mix chia seeds, almond milk, and honey in a jar or bowl. Stir well, cover, and refrigerate overnight. In the morning, top with your favorite fruits or nuts before serving.

2. **Whole Grain Toast with Nut Butter**
   - o *Ingredients:* 2 slices whole grain bread, 2 tablespoons nut butter (such as almond or peanut butter), sliced fruits for topping.
   - o *Instructions:* Toast the bread slices until golden brown. Spread nut butter evenly on each slice and top with sliced fruits for added flavor and nutrition.

3. **Fruit and Yogurt Bowl**
   - o *Ingredients:* 1/2 cup Greek yogurt, 1/2 cup mixed fruits (such as berries, banana slices, or apple chunks), 1 tablespoon honey or maple syrup, granola or nuts for crunch.
   - o *Instructions:* In a bowl, layer Greek yogurt, mixed fruits, and granola or nuts. Drizzle with honey or maple syrup for sweetness.

4. **Microwave Egg Muffin**
   - o *Ingredients:* 2 eggs, 1/4 cup chopped vegetables (such as bell peppers, onions, or spinach), 2 tablespoons shredded cheese, salt, and pepper to taste.
   - o *Instructions:* Beat eggs in a microwave-safe mug or bowl. Stir in chopped vegetables, cheese, salt, and pepper. Microwave on high for 1-2 minutes until eggs are fully cooked. Enjoy as is or on a whole grain English muffin for a breakfast sandwich.

5. **Banana and Peanut Butter Roll-Ups**
   - o *Ingredients:* 1 whole grain tortilla, 1 banana, 2 tablespoons peanut butter, honey for drizzling (optional).

- o *Instructions:* Spread peanut butter evenly on the tortilla. Place a peeled banana on one end and roll it up tightly. Slice into bite-sized pieces and drizzle with honey if desired. Enjoy as a quick and portable breakfast option.

These breakfast options are not only delicious but also packed with nutrients to kickstart your day on the right note. Feel free to mix and match ingredients based on your preferences and dietary requirements.

## 8. Lunch

# Brain-Boosting Salads

1. **Mediterranean Quinoa Salad**
   - o *Ingredients:* 1 cup cooked quinoa, 1/2 cup cherry tomatoes (halved), 1/4 cup diced cucumber, 1/4 cup diced red onion, 1/4 cup crumbled feta cheese, 2 tablespoons chopped Kalamata olives, 2 tablespoons olive oil, juice of 1 lemon, salt, and pepper to taste.
   - o *Instructions:* In a bowl, combine cooked quinoa, cherry tomatoes, cucumber, red onion, feta cheese, and olives. Drizzle with olive oil and lemon juice. Season with salt and pepper. Toss gently to combine.
2. **Asian-Inspired Chicken Salad**
   - o *Ingredients:* 2 cups mixed greens, 1 cooked chicken breast (sliced), 1/4 cup shredded carrots, 1/4 cup shredded red cabbage, 1/4 cup edamame, 1/4 cup sliced almonds, 2 tablespoons sesame ginger dressing.
   - o *Instructions:* Arrange mixed greens on a plate. Top with sliced chicken breast, shredded carrots, shredded

red cabbage, edamame, and sliced almonds. Drizzle with sesame ginger dressing before serving.

3. **Kale and Avocado Salad**
   o *Ingredients:* 2 cups chopped kale, 1/2 avocado (diced), 1/4 cup sliced strawberries, 2 tablespoons crumbled goat cheese, 2 tablespoons balsamic vinaigrette, 1 tablespoon sunflower seeds.
   o *Instructions:* Massage kale with balsamic vinaigrette to soften. Top with diced avocado, sliced strawberries, crumbled goat cheese, and sunflower seeds. Toss gently to combine.

4. **Tuna and White Bean Salad**
   o *Ingredients:* 1 can tuna (drained), 1 can white beans (drained and rinsed), 1/4 cup diced red onion, 1/4 cup chopped parsley, 2 tablespoons olive oil, juice of 1 lemon, salt, and pepper to taste.
   o *Instructions:* In a bowl, combine tuna, white beans, red onion, and parsley. Drizzle with olive oil and lemon juice. Season with salt and pepper. Mix well and serve chilled.

5. **Roasted Vegetable Quinoa Salad**
   o *Ingredients:* 1 cup cooked quinoa, 1 cup roasted vegetables (such as bell peppers, zucchini, and eggplant), 1/4 cup crumbled feta cheese, 2 tablespoons balsamic vinaigrette, fresh basil leaves for garnish.
   o *Instructions:* In a bowl, combine cooked quinoa, roasted vegetables, and crumbled feta cheese. Drizzle with balsamic vinaigrette and toss gently to combine. Garnish with fresh basil leaves before serving.

# Hearty Soups and Stews

1. **Vegetable Lentil Soup**
   - *Ingredients:* 1 cup lentils, 4 cups vegetable broth, 1 onion (diced), 2 carrots (diced), 2 celery stalks (diced), 2 cloves garlic (minced), 1 can diced tomatoes, 1 teaspoon cumin, 1 teaspoon paprika, salt, and pepper to taste.
   - *Instructions:* In a large pot, combine lentils, vegetable broth, onion, carrots, celery, garlic, and diced tomatoes. Season with cumin, paprika, salt, and pepper. Bring to a boil, then reduce heat and simmer for 20-25 minutes until lentils are tender.

2. **Chicken and Vegetable Stew**
   - *Ingredients:* 2 chicken breasts (cut into cubes), 4 cups chicken broth, 2 potatoes (diced), 2 carrots (sliced), 1 onion (diced), 2 cloves garlic (minced), 1 teaspoon thyme, 1 teaspoon rosemary, salt, and pepper to taste.
   - *Instructions:* In a large pot, heat olive oil over medium heat. Add chicken cubes and cook until browned. Add diced potatoes, carrots, onion, and garlic. Cook for 5 minutes, then add chicken broth, thyme, rosemary, salt, and pepper. Simmer for 20-25 minutes until vegetables are tender and chicken is cooked through.

3. **Tomato Basil Soup**
   - *Ingredients:* 4 cups tomatoes (diced), 1 onion (diced), 2 cloves garlic (minced), 2 cups vegetable broth, 1/4 cup fresh basil leaves, 1/4 cup heavy cream, salt, and pepper to taste.
   - *Instructions:* In a large pot, sauté onion and garlic in olive oil until soft. Add diced tomatoes and vegetable

broth. Simmer for 15-20 minutes. Stir in fresh basil leaves and heavy cream. Use an immersion blender to blend until smooth. Season with salt and pepper before serving.

4. **Minestrone Soup**
   - *Ingredients:* 4 cups vegetable broth, 1 can diced tomatoes, 1 onion (diced), 2 carrots (diced), 2 celery stalks (diced), 1 zucchini (diced), 1 cup cooked pasta, 1 can kidney beans (drained and rinsed), 1 teaspoon Italian seasoning, salt, and pepper to taste.
   - *Instructions:* In a large pot, combine vegetable broth, diced tomatoes, onion, carrots, celery, zucchini, cooked pasta, and kidney beans. Season with Italian seasoning, salt, and pepper. Bring to a boil, then reduce heat and simmer for 20-25 minutes until vegetables are tender.

5. **Butternut Squash and Apple Soup**
   - *Ingredients:* 1 butternut squash (peeled, seeded, and diced), 2 apples (peeled, cored, and diced), 1 onion (diced), 2 cloves garlic (minced), 4 cups vegetable broth, 1/2 teaspoon cinnamon, 1/4 teaspoon nutmeg, salt, and pepper to taste.
   - *Instructions:* In a large pot, sauté onion and garlic in olive oil until soft. Add diced butternut squash, apples, vegetable broth, cinnamon, nutmeg, salt, and pepper. Simmer for 20-25 minutes until squash and apples are tender. Use an immersion blender to blend until smooth. Serve hot.

# Simple Sandwiches and Wraps

1. **Turkey and Avocado Wrap**
   - *Ingredients:* 1 whole grain wrap, 3 slices deli turkey, 1/4 avocado (sliced), 1/4 cup mixed greens, 1 tablespoon hummus.
   - *Instructions:* Spread hummus evenly on the wrap. Layer with turkey slices, avocado slices, and mixed greens. Roll up tightly and slice in half.
2. **Caprese Sandwich**
   - *Ingredients:* 2 slices whole grain bread, 2 slices mozzarella cheese, 1 tomato (sliced), fresh basil leaves, balsamic glaze.

*Instructions:* Layer mozzarella cheese, tomato slices, and fresh basil leaves on one slice of bread. Drizzle with balsamic glaze and top with the other slice of bread. Press gently to form a sandwich. Cut in half and serve.

3. **Grilled Chicken Caesar Wrap**
   - *Ingredients:* 1 whole grain wrap, 1 grilled chicken breast (sliced), 1/4 cup romaine lettuce (chopped), 2 tablespoons Caesar dressing, 1 tablespoon grated Parmesan cheese.
   - *Instructions:* Lay the wrap flat and layer with grilled chicken slices and chopped romaine lettuce. Drizzle with Caesar dressing and sprinkle with grated Parmesan cheese. Roll up tightly and slice before serving.
4. **Veggie Hummus Wrap**
   - *Ingredients:* 1 whole grain wrap, 2 tablespoons hummus, 1/4 cup sliced cucumber, 1/4 cup shredded

carrots, 1/4 cup sliced bell peppers, 1/4 cup mixed greens.

- *Instructions:* Spread hummus evenly on the wrap. Layer with sliced cucumber, shredded carrots, sliced bell peppers, and mixed greens. Roll up tightly and slice in half.

5. **Tuna Salad Sandwich**
   - *Ingredients:* 2 slices whole grain bread, 1 can tuna (drained), 2 tablespoons Greek yogurt, 1 tablespoon diced celery, 1 tablespoon diced red onion, salt, and pepper to taste.
   - *Instructions:* In a bowl, mix tuna, Greek yogurt, diced celery, and diced red onion. Season with salt and pepper. Spread tuna salad evenly on one slice of bread. Top with the other slice of bread to form a sandwich. Cut in half and serve.

These lunch options provide a balance of nutrients and flavors to keep you satisfied and energized throughout the day. Feel free to customize them with your favorite ingredients and sauces.

## 9. Dinner

# Balanced Main Courses

1. **Grilled Salmon with Quinoa and Asparagus**
   - *Ingredients:*
     - 2 salmon fillets
     - 1 cup cooked quinoa
     - 1 bunch asparagus, trimmed

- 2 tablespoons olive oil
- 1 lemon, sliced
- Salt and pepper to taste

- o *Instructions:*

  - Preheat grill to medium-high heat.
  - Season salmon fillets with salt, pepper, and a drizzle of olive oil.
  - Place salmon fillets and asparagus on the grill. Cook salmon for 4-5 minutes per side, or until cooked through, and cook asparagus for 3-4 minutes, turning occasionally.
  - Serve grilled salmon and asparagus over cooked quinoa. Garnish with lemon slices before serving.

2. **Stuffed Bell Peppers with Ground Turkey**
   - o *Ingredients:*

     - 4 bell peppers, halved and seeds removed
     - 1 pound ground turkey
     - 1 cup cooked quinoa
     - 1 onion, diced
     - 2 cloves garlic, minced
     - 1 can diced tomatoes
     - 1 teaspoon Italian seasoning
     - Salt and pepper to taste

   - o *Instructions:*

     - Preheat oven to 375°F (190°C).
     - In a skillet, cook ground turkey, onion, and garlic until turkey is browned and onions are translucent. Drain any excess fat.

- Stir in cooked quinoa, diced tomatoes, Italian seasoning, salt, and pepper. Cook for an additional 5 minutes.
- Spoon turkey mixture into halved bell peppers. Place stuffed peppers in a baking dish.
- Cover with foil and bake for 25-30 minutes, or until peppers are tender. Remove foil and bake for an additional 5 minutes. Serve hot.

3. **Lemon Garlic Chicken with Roasted Vegetables**
   - *Ingredients:*

     - 4 boneless, skinless chicken breasts
     - 1 pound baby potatoes, halved
     - 1 bunch broccoli, cut into florets
     - 4 cloves garlic, minced
     - 2 tablespoons olive oil
     - 1 lemon, juiced and zested
     - 1 teaspoon dried thyme
     - Salt and pepper to taste
   - *Instructions:*

     - Preheat oven to 400°F (200°C).
     - In a small bowl, whisk together minced garlic, olive oil, lemon juice, lemon zest, dried thyme, salt, and pepper.
     - Place chicken breasts in a baking dish. Arrange halved baby potatoes and broccoli around the chicken.
     - Pour the lemon garlic mixture over the chicken and vegetables, ensuring everything is evenly coated.

- Bake for 25-30 minutes, or until chicken is cooked through and vegetables are tender. Serve hot.

4. **Beef Stir-Fry with Brown Rice**
    o *Ingredients:*

    - 1 pound beef sirloin, thinly sliced
    - 2 cups mixed vegetables (such as bell peppers, broccoli, and snap peas)
    - 3 cloves garlic, minced
    - 2 tablespoons soy sauce
    - 1 tablespoon oyster sauce
    - 1 tablespoon sesame oil
    - 2 cups cooked brown rice
    - Green onions, sliced, for garnish

    o *Instructions:*

    - In a large skillet or wok, heat sesame oil over medium-high heat. Add minced garlic and cook until fragrant.
    - Add sliced beef to the skillet and cook until browned.
    - Stir in mixed vegetables and cook until tender-crisp.
    - Add soy sauce and oyster sauce to the skillet, stirring to combine.
    - Serve beef stir-fry over cooked brown rice. Garnish with sliced green onions before serving.

5. **Pasta Primavera**
    o *Ingredients:*

    - 8 ounces whole wheat pasta

- 2 tablespoons olive oil
- 2 cloves garlic, minced
- 2 cups mixed vegetables (such as bell peppers, cherry tomatoes, zucchini, and mushrooms), sliced
- 1/4 cup grated Parmesan cheese
- Salt and pepper to taste

- *Instructions:*

  - Cook pasta according to package instructions. Drain and set aside.
  - In a large skillet, heat olive oil over medium heat. Add minced garlic and cook until fragrant.
  - Add mixed vegetables to the skillet and cook until tender.
  - Toss cooked pasta with the vegetables in the skillet. Season with salt and pepper.
  - Serve pasta primavera hot, garnished with grated Parmesan cheese.

# Vegetarian and Vegan Options

1. **Vegetable Stir-Fry with Tofu**
   - *Ingredients:*
     - 1 block extra-firm tofu, pressed and cubed
     - 2 tablespoons soy sauce
     - 1 tablespoon cornstarch
     - 2 tablespoons vegetable oil
     - 2 cups mixed vegetables (such as bell peppers, broccoli, carrots, and snap peas)
     - 3 cloves garlic, minced

- 1 tablespoon fresh ginger, grated
- Cooked rice or noodles for serving

- *Instructions:*

  - In a bowl, toss cubed tofu with soy sauce and cornstarch until evenly coated.
  - Heat vegetable oil in a large skillet or wok over medium-high heat. Add tofu cubes and cook until golden brown on all sides. Remove tofu from the skillet and set aside.
  - In the same skillet, add more oil if needed and sauté minced garlic and grated ginger until fragrant.
  - Add mixed vegetables to the skillet and stir-fry until tender-crisp.
  - Return cooked tofu to the skillet and toss everything together. Serve vegetable stir-fry over cooked rice or noodles.

2. **Chickpea and Vegetable Curry**
   - *Ingredients:*

     - 1 tablespoon coconut oil
     - 1 onion, diced
     - 2 cloves garlic, minced
     - 1 tablespoon curry powder
     - 1 can chickpeas, drained and rinsed
     - 1 can diced tomatoes
     - 1 can coconut milk
     - 2 cups mixed vegetables (such as cauliflower, bell peppers, and spinach)
     - Cooked rice for serving
   - *Instructions:*

- In a large pot, heat coconut oil over medium heat. Add diced onion and minced garlic, and cook until softened.
- Stir in curry powder and cook for another minute until fragrant.
- Add chickpeas, diced tomatoes, coconut milk, and mixed vegetables to the pot. Stir to combine.
- Bring the curry to a simmer and cook for 15-20 minutes, or until vegetables are tender.
- Serve chickpea and vegetable curry hot over cooked rice.

3. **Eggplant Parmesan**

- *Ingredients:*
  - 1 large eggplant, sliced into rounds
  - 1 cup breadcrumbs (or almond flour for gluten-free option)
  - 2 eggs (or flaxseed eggs for vegan option)
  - 1 cup marinara sauce
  - 1 cup shredded mozzarella cheese (or vegan cheese)
  - 1/4 cup grated Parmesan cheese (or nutritional yeast for vegan option)
  - Fresh basil leaves for garnish
  - Salt and pepper to taste
- *Instructions:*

  - Preheat oven to 400°F (200°C). Line a baking sheet with parchment paper.
  - In one shallow dish, beat the eggs. In another shallow dish, place breadcrumbs (or almond flour).

- o Dip each eggplant slice into the beaten eggs, then coat with breadcrumbs (or almond flour). Place the coated eggplant slices on the prepared baking sheet.
- o Bake eggplant slices in the preheated oven for 15-20 minutes, or until golden brown and crispy.
- o Remove from the oven and reduce the oven temperature to 350°F (175°C). Spread a thin layer of marinara sauce in the bottom of a baking dish.
- o Arrange half of the baked eggplant slices in the baking dish. Top with more marinara sauce, shredded mozzarella cheese, and grated Parmesan cheese. Repeat the layers with the remaining eggplant slices and toppings.
- o Bake eggplant Parmesan in the oven for 20-25 minutes, or until the cheese is melted and bubbly.
- o Garnish with fresh basil leaves before serving.

4. **Mushroom Risotto**
   - o *Ingredients:*
     - 1 cup Arborio rice
     - 4 cups vegetable broth
     - 1 onion, finely chopped
     - 2 cloves garlic, minced
     - 1 cup mushrooms, sliced
     - 1/2 cup dry white wine (optional)
     - 1/4 cup grated Parmesan cheese (or nutritional yeast for vegan option)
     - 2 tablespoons olive oil
     - Salt and pepper to taste
   - o *Instructions:*

     - In a saucepan, heat vegetable broth over low heat and keep warm.

- In a separate large pot, heat olive oil over medium heat. Add chopped onion and minced garlic, and sauté until softened.
- Add Arborio rice to the pot and cook, stirring constantly, for 1-2 minutes until lightly toasted.
- If using white wine, pour it into the pot and stir until absorbed.
- Begin adding warm vegetable broth to the rice mixture, one ladleful at a time, stirring frequently. Wait until the broth is absorbed before adding more.
- Continue this process until the rice is creamy and tender, about 20-25 minutes.
- In the last few minutes of cooking, stir in sliced mushrooms and cook until tender.
- Remove the risotto from heat and stir in grated Parmesan cheese (or nutritional yeast). Season with salt and pepper to taste before serving.

5. **Vegetable Fajitas**
   - *Ingredients:*

     - 1 bell pepper, sliced
     - 1 onion, sliced
     - 1 zucchini, sliced
     - 1 cup mushrooms, sliced
     - 2 tablespoons olive oil
     - 2 tablespoons fajita seasoning
     - 8 small whole wheat tortillas
     - Optional toppings: avocado, salsa, Greek yogurt (or sour cream), shredded cheese (or vegan cheese)

o *Instructions:*

- Heat olive oil in a large skillet over medium-high heat.
- Add sliced bell pepper, onion, zucchini, and mushrooms to the skillet. Sprinkle fajita seasoning over the vegetables and toss to coat.
- Cook vegetables, stirring occasionally, until they are tender and slightly charred, about 8-10 minutes.
- Warm whole wheat tortillas in a separate skillet or in the microwave.
- Spoon cooked vegetables onto warmed tortillas. Add optional toppings such as avocado, salsa, Greek yogurt (or sour cream), and shredded cheese (or vegan cheese).
- Roll up the tortillas and serve vegetable fajitas hot.

# Slow Cooker Recipes for Convenience

1. **Slow Cooker Chicken and Vegetable Curry**
   o *Ingredients:*
   - 1 pound chicken breasts, cut into cubes
   - 2 cups mixed vegetables (such as carrots, bell peppers, and peas)
   - 1 onion, diced
   - 2 cloves garlic, minced
   - 1 can coconut milk
   - 1/4 cup curry paste
   - 2 tablespoons soy sauce
   - Cooked rice for serving

o *Instructions:*

- In a slow cooker, combine chicken cubes, mixed vegetables, diced onion, minced garlic, coconut milk, curry paste, and soy sauce.
- Stir to combine all ingredients.
- Cover and cook on low heat for 6-8 hours or high heat for 3-4 hours, until chicken is cooked through and vegetables are tender.
- Serve chicken and vegetable curry over cooked rice.

2. **Slow Cooker Lentil Soup**
   - *Ingredients:*

     - 1 cup dried lentils
     - 4 cups vegetable broth
     - 1 onion, diced
     - 2 carrots, diced
     - 2 celery stalks, diced
     - 2 cloves garlic, minced
     - 1 can diced tomatoes
     - 1 teaspoon dried thyme
     - Salt and pepper to taste

   - *Instructions:*

     - Rinse dried lentils under cold water and drain.
     - In a slow cooker, combine lentils, vegetable broth, diced onion, diced carrots, diced celery, minced garlic, diced tomatoes, dried thyme, salt, and pepper.
     - Stir to combine all ingredients.
     - Cover and cook on low heat for 6-8 hours or high heat for 3-4 hours, until lentils are tender.
     - Serve lentil soup hot, garnished with fresh parsley if desired.

3. **Slow Cooker Beef Stew**
   - *Ingredients:*

     - 1 pound beef stew meat, cubed
     - 4 cups beef broth
     - 2 potatoes, diced
     - 2 carrots, sliced
     - 1 onion, diced
     - 2 cloves garlic, minced

- 1 teaspoon dried thyme
- 1 teaspoon dried rosemary
- Salt and pepper to taste

o *Instructions:*

1. In a slow cooker, combine beef stew meat, beef broth, diced potatoes, sliced carrots, diced onion, minced garlic, dried thyme, dried rosemary, salt, and pepper.
2. Stir to combine all ingredients.
3. Cover and cook on low heat for 6-8 hours or high heat for 3-4 hours, until beef is tender.
4. Serve beef stew hot, garnished with chopped fresh parsley if desired.

4. **Slow Cooker Vegetarian Chili**
   o *Ingredients:*
   - 1 can kidney beans, drained and rinsed
   - 1 can black beans, drained and rinsed
   - 1 can diced tomatoes
   - 1 onion, diced
   - 2 cloves garlic, minced
   - 1 bell pepper, diced
   - 1 cup corn kernels (fresh or frozen)
   - 1 tablespoon chili powder
   - 1 teaspoon cumin
   - Salt and pepper to taste
   o *Instructions:*

   - In a slow cooker, combine kidney beans, black beans, diced tomatoes, diced onion, minced garlic, diced bell pepper, corn kernels, chili powder, cumin, salt, and pepper.

- Stir to combine all ingredients.
- Cover and cook on low heat for 6-8 hours or high heat for 3-4 hours.
- Serve vegetarian chili hot, garnished with shredded cheese, chopped green onions, and a dollop of sour cream if desired.

5. **Slow Cooker Vegetable Lasagna**
   - *Ingredients:*

     - 9 lasagna noodles, uncooked
     - 2 cups marinara sauce
     - 2 cups mixed vegetables (such as zucchini, bell peppers, mushrooms, and spinach), sliced
     - 2 cups ricotta cheese (or cottage cheese)
     - 1 cup shredded mozzarella cheese
     - 1/4 cup grated Parmesan cheese
     - 1 teaspoon dried basil
     - 1 teaspoon dried oregano
     - Salt and pepper to taste

   - *Instructions:*

     - In a bowl, mix together ricotta cheese, shredded mozzarella cheese, grated Parmesan cheese, dried basil, dried oregano, salt, and pepper.
     - Spread a thin layer of marinara sauce in the bottom of the slow cooker.
     - Arrange 3 lasagna noodles over the marinara sauce, breaking noodles to fit if necessary.
     - Top noodles with half of the ricotta cheese mixture and half of the mixed vegetables.

- Repeat layers with marinara sauce, lasagna noodles, remaining ricotta cheese mixture, and remaining mixed vegetables.
- Finish with a final layer of marinara sauce and sprinkle with additional shredded mozzarella cheese and grated Parmesan cheese.
- Cover and cook on low heat for 4-6 hours, or until noodles are tender and cheese is melted and bubbly.
- Serve vegetable lasagna hot, garnished with fresh basil leaves if desired.

These slow cooker recipes offer convenience and flavor, allowing you to enjoy a delicious and nutritious dinner with minimal effort. Adjust the ingredients and seasonings according to your preferences for a personalized touch.

## 10. Snacks and Sides

# Healthy Snack Ideas

1. **Greek Yogurt with Berries**
   - *Ingredients:*
     - 1/2 cup Greek yogurt
     - 1/4 cup mixed berries (such as strawberries, blueberries, and raspberries)
     - 1 tablespoon honey (optional)
   - *Instructions:*
     - Spoon Greek yogurt into a bowl or cup.
     - Top with mixed berries.
     - Drizzle with honey if desired.

- Enjoy this protein-packed and antioxidant-rich snack.

2. **Homemade Trail Mix**
   o *Ingredients:*

   - 1/4 cup almonds
   - 1/4 cup cashews
   - 1/4 cup dried cranberries
   - 1/4 cup dark chocolate chips
   - 1/4 cup pumpkin seeds

   o *Instructions:*

   - Combine all ingredients in a bowl and mix well.
   - Portion into individual snack bags for a convenient grab-and-go option.
   - This trail mix provides a balance of healthy fats, protein, and carbohydrates for sustained energy.

3. **Vegetable Sticks with Hummus**
   o *Ingredients:*

   - Carrot sticks
   - Celery sticks
   - Cucumber slices
   - Cherry tomatoes
   - Hummus for dipping

   o *Instructions:*

   - Wash and cut vegetables into sticks or slices.
   - Serve with hummus for a crunchy and satisfying snack.

- This snack is rich in fiber, vitamins, and minerals, perfect for keeping you full and energized between meals.

4. **Apple Slices with Peanut Butter**
   - *Ingredients:*

     - 1 apple, sliced
     - 2 tablespoons peanut butter (or almond butter for a variation)

   - *Instructions:*

     - Slice the apple into thin wedges.
     - Spread peanut butter on each apple slice.
     - Enjoy the combination of sweet and savory flavors, along with a boost of protein and fiber.

5. **Roasted Chickpeas**
   - *Ingredients:*

     - 1 can chickpeas, drained and rinsed
     - 1 tablespoon olive oil
     - 1 teaspoon smoked paprika
     - 1/2 teaspoon garlic powder
     - 1/2 teaspoon cumin
     - Salt to taste

   - *Instructions:*

     - Preheat oven to 400°F (200°C).
     - Pat dry the chickpeas with a paper towel to remove excess moisture.
     - In a bowl, toss chickpeas with olive oil, smoked paprika, garlic powder, cumin, and salt until evenly coated.

- Spread chickpeas in a single layer on a baking sheet.
- Roast in the preheated oven for 25-30 minutes, or until chickpeas are crispy.
- Let cool before enjoying this crunchy and protein-rich snack.

# Nutritious Side Dishes

1. **Quinoa Salad**
   - *Ingredients:*
     - 1 cup cooked quinoa
     - 1/2 cup diced cucumber
     - 1/2 cup diced bell pepper (any color)
     - 1/4 cup chopped fresh parsley
     - 2 tablespoons olive oil
     - 1 tablespoon lemon juice
     - Salt and pepper to taste
   - *Instructions:*
     - In a bowl, combine cooked quinoa, diced cucumber, diced bell pepper, and chopped fresh parsley.
     - Drizzle with olive oil and lemon juice. Season with salt and pepper.
     - Toss until well combined.
     - Serve as a refreshing and nutritious side dish to complement any meal.

2. **Steamed Broccoli with Garlic**
   - *Ingredients:*
     - 2 cups broccoli florets

- 2 cloves garlic, minced
- 1 tablespoon olive oil
- Salt and pepper to taste

o *Instructions:*

- Steam broccoli florets until tender-crisp, about 5-7 minutes.
- In a skillet, heat olive oil over medium heat.
- Add minced garlic and sauté until fragrant, about 1 minute.
- Add steamed broccoli to the skillet and toss to coat with garlic-infused oil.
- Season with salt and pepper.
- Serve as a healthy and flavorful side dish.

3. **Baked Sweet Potato Wedges**
   - *Ingredients:*

     - 2 medium sweet potatoes, scrubbed and cut into wedges
     - 2 tablespoons olive oil
     - 1 teaspoon smoked paprika
     - 1/2 teaspoon garlic powder
     - 1/2 teaspoon cumin
     - Salt and pepper to taste

   - *Instructions:*

     - Preheat oven to 425°F (220°C).
     - In a large bowl, toss sweet potato wedges with olive oil, smoked paprika, garlic powder, cumin, salt, and pepper until evenly coated.
     - Arrange sweet potato wedges in a single layer on a baking sheet.
     - Bake in the preheated oven for 25-30 minutes, flipping halfway through, until golden brown and crispy.
     - Serve as a nutritious and satisfying side dish or snack.

4. **Quinoa and Vegetable Stir-Fry**
   - *Ingredients:*

     - 1 cup cooked quinoa
     - 2 cups mixed vegetables (such as bell peppers, broccoli, carrots, and snap peas), sliced
     - 2 cloves garlic, minced
     - 2 tablespoons soy sauce
     - 1 tablespoon sesame oil
     - 1 tablespoon rice vinegar

- 1 teaspoon ginger, grated
- Sesame seeds for garnish

- o *Instructions:*

  - In a skillet or wok, heat sesame oil over medium-high heat.
  - Add minced garlic and grated ginger, and sauté until fragrant.
  - Add mixed vegetables to the skillet and stir-fry until tender-crisp.
  - Stir in cooked quinoa, soy sauce, and rice vinegar. Cook until heated through.
  - Serve quinoa and vegetable stir-fry hot, garnished with sesame seeds.

5. **Caprese Salad**
   - o *Ingredients:*

     - 2 large tomatoes, sliced
     - 1 ball fresh mozzarella cheese, sliced
     - Fresh basil leaves
     - Balsamic glaze
     - Salt and pepper to taste

   - o *Instructions:*
     1. Arrange tomato slices and fresh mozzarella slices on a serving platter, alternating between them.
     2. Tuck fresh basil leaves between the tomato and mozzarella slices.
     3. Drizzle balsamic glaze over the salad.
     4. Season with salt and pepper to taste.
     5. Serve as a light and refreshing side dish or appetizer.

# Quick Bites for Energy

1.  **Energy Bites**
    o   *Ingredients:*
        - 1 cup rolled oats
        - 1/2 cup nut butter (such as peanut butter or almond butter)
        - 1/4 cup honey or maple syrup
        - 1/4 cup ground flaxseed
        - 1/4 cup mini chocolate chips
        - 1 teaspoon vanilla extract
    o   *Instructions:*

        - In a large bowl, mix together rolled oats, nut butter, honey or maple syrup, ground flaxseed, mini chocolate chips, and vanilla extract until well combined.
        - Roll the mixture into small balls, about 1 inch in diameter.
        - Place energy bites on a baking sheet lined with parchment paper.
        - Chill in the refrigerator for at least 30 minutes before serving.
        - Enjoy these nutritious and portable snacks for a quick energy boost.

2.  **Apple Sandwiches with Almond Butter**
    o   *Ingredients:*

        - 1 apple, cored and sliced into rounds
        - 2 tablespoons almond butter (or any nut or seed butter)

- Granola, chopped nuts, or dried fruit for topping (optional)
  - *Instructions:*

    - Spread almond butter onto one apple slice.
    - Top with another apple slice to form a sandwich.
    - Optional: Roll the edges of the apple sandwich in granola, chopped nuts, or dried fruit for added texture and flavor.
    - Repeat with remaining apple slices and almond butter.
    - Enjoy these apple sandwiches as a quick and satisfying snack.

3. **Cucumber Slices with Cottage Cheese**
   - *Ingredients:*

     - 1 cucumber, sliced into rounds
     - 1/2 cup cottage cheese
     - Everything bagel seasoning for topping (optional)
   - *Instructions:*

     - Place cucumber slices on a serving plate.
     - Spoon cottage cheese onto each cucumber slice.
     - Optional: Sprinkle everything bagel seasoning on top of the cottage cheese for added flavor.
     - Serve these cucumber slices with cottage cheese as a refreshing and protein-rich snack.

4. **Whole Grain Crackers with Guacamole**
   - *Ingredients:*

- Whole grain crackers
- 1 ripe avocado, mashed
- 1 tablespoon lime juice
- 1/4 teaspoon garlic powder
- Salt and pepper to taste

o *Instructions:*

- In a bowl, mash the ripe avocado with lime juice, garlic powder, salt, and pepper until smooth.
- Spread guacamole onto whole grain crackers.
- Serve these crackers with guacamole as a satisfying and nutrient-packed snack.

5. **Hard-Boiled Eggs with Hummus**

o *Ingredients:*

- Hard-boiled eggs, peeled
- Hummus for dipping

o *Instructions:*

- Slice hard-boiled eggs in half lengthwise.
- Serve with hummus for dipping.
- Enjoy these hard-boiled eggs with hummus as a protein-rich and filling snack option.

These quick bites provide energy and nutrition on-the-go, perfect for refueling between meals or satisfying mid-afternoon cravings. Enjoy them as standalone snacks or combine them for a balanced and flavorful snack platter.

## 11. Desserts and Treats

## Low-Sugar Dessert Options

1. **Chia Seed Pudding**
   - *Ingredients:*
     - 1/4 cup chia seeds
     - 1 cup almond milk (or any milk of choice)
     - 1 tablespoon maple syrup (or honey)
     - 1/2 teaspoon vanilla extract
     - Fresh fruit for topping (such as berries or sliced bananas)
   - *Instructions:*

     - In a bowl or jar, mix together chia seeds, almond milk, maple syrup (or honey), and vanilla extract.
     - Stir well to combine.
     - Cover and refrigerate for at least 2 hours, or overnight, until the chia pudding thickens.
     - Serve chilled, topped with fresh fruit.
     - Enjoy this low-sugar dessert option for a satisfying and nutritious treat.

2. **Baked Apples**
   - *Ingredients:*

     - 2 apples, cored
     - 2 tablespoons chopped nuts (such as walnuts or almonds)
     - 1 tablespoon raisins or dried cranberries
     - 1/2 teaspoon cinnamon
     - 1 teaspoon honey (optional)
   - *Instructions:*

     - Preheat oven to 375°F (190°C).

- In a small bowl, mix together chopped nuts, raisins or dried cranberries, cinnamon, and honey (if using).
- Stuff each cored apple with the nut mixture.
- Place stuffed apples in a baking dish and bake in the preheated oven for 25-30 minutes, or until apples are tender.
- Serve baked apples warm, optionally topped with a dollop of Greek yogurt or a sprinkle of granola.

3. **Frozen Yogurt Bark**
   - *Ingredients:*

     - 2 cups Greek yogurt
     - 2 tablespoons honey or maple syrup
     - 1/2 cup mixed berries (such as strawberries, blueberries, and raspberries)
     - 2 tablespoons chopped nuts (such as almonds or pistachios)
   - *Instructions:*

     - In a bowl, mix together Greek yogurt and honey or maple syrup until smooth.
     - Line a baking sheet with parchment paper.
     - Spread the yogurt mixture evenly onto the parchment paper, about 1/4 inch thick.
     - Sprinkle mixed berries and chopped nuts over the yogurt.
     - Freeze yogurt bark for 2-3 hours, or until firm.
     - Break the frozen yogurt bark into pieces and serve immediately.
     - Enjoy this refreshing and low-sugar dessert option straight from the freezer.

4. **Dark Chocolate Covered Strawberries**
   - *Ingredients:*

     - Fresh strawberries, rinsed and dried
     - Dark chocolate chips

   - *Instructions:*

     - Line a baking sheet with parchment paper.
     - In a microwave-safe bowl, melt dark chocolate chips in 30-second intervals, stirring between each interval, until smooth.
     - Dip each strawberry into the melted chocolate, covering about half of the strawberry.
     - Place chocolate-covered strawberries on the prepared baking sheet.
     - Refrigerate for 15-20 minutes, or until the chocolate is set.
     - Serve dark chocolate covered strawberries as a decadent and low-sugar dessert option.

5. **Coconut Date Balls**
   - *Ingredients:*

     - 1 cup pitted dates
     - 1/2 cup shredded coconut
     - 1/4 cup almond flour
     - 1/4 cup chopped nuts (such as pecans or cashews)
     - 1 tablespoon coconut oil
     - 1/2 teaspoon vanilla extract

   - *Instructions:*

- In a food processor, combine pitted dates, shredded coconut, almond flour, chopped nuts, coconut oil, and vanilla extract.
- Process until the mixture comes together and forms a sticky dough.
- Roll the dough into small balls, about 1 inch in diameter.
- Optional: Roll coconut date balls in additional shredded coconut for coating.
- Refrigerate coconut date balls for at least 30 minutes before serving.
- Enjoy these naturally sweet and satisfying treats as a guilt-free dessert option.

# Healthy Baking Recipes

1. **Banana Oatmeal Cookies**
   - *Ingredients:*
     - 2 ripe bananas, mashed
     - 1 1/2 cups rolled oats
     - 1/4 cup almond butter (or any nut or seed butter)
     - 1/4 cup dark chocolate chips (optional)
     - 1/4 teaspoon cinnamon
     - 1/4 teaspoon vanilla extract
   - *Instructions:*

     - Preheat oven to 350°F (175°C). Line a baking sheet with parchment paper.
     - In a bowl, combine mashed bananas, rolled oats, almond butter, dark chocolate chips (if using), cinnamon, and vanilla extract.
     - Mix until all ingredients are well combined.
     - Drop spoonfuls of the cookie dough onto the prepared baking sheet.
     - Flatten each cookie with the back of a spoon.
     - Bake in the preheated oven for 12-15 minutes, or until cookies are golden brown.
     - Let cool before enjoying these soft and chewy banana oatmeal cookies.

2. **Sweet Potato Brownies**
   - *Ingredients:*

     - 1 cup mashed sweet potato
     - 1/2 cup almond butter (or any nut or seed butter)

- 1/4 cup maple syrup
- 1/4 cup cocoa powder
- 1 teaspoon vanilla extract
- 1/4 teaspoon baking soda
- 1/4 cup dark chocolate chips (optional)

o *Instructions:*

- Preheat oven to 350°F (175°C). Grease a baking dish with coconut oil or line with parchment paper.
- In a bowl, mix together mashed sweet potato, almond butter, maple syrup, cocoa powder, vanilla extract, and baking soda until smooth.
- Fold in dark chocolate chips if desired.
- Spread the brownie batter evenly into the prepared baking dish.
- Bake in the preheated oven for 25-30 minutes, or until the edges are set and a toothpick inserted into the center comes out clean.
- Let cool before slicing into squares.
- Enjoy these indulgent yet healthy sweet potato brownies as a guilt-free treat.

3. **Zucchini Bread**

- *Ingredients:*
  o 2 cups shredded zucchini
  o 2 cups almond flour
  o 1/2 cup coconut sugar
  o 1/4 cup coconut oil, melted
  o 2 eggs
  o 1 teaspoon vanilla extract
  o 1 teaspoon cinnamon
  o 1/2 teaspoon baking powder

- o 1/2 teaspoon baking soda
- o 1/4 teaspoon salt
- *Instructions:*

1. Preheat oven to 350°F (175°C). Grease a loaf pan with coconut oil or line with parchment paper.
2. In a large bowl, combine shredded zucchini, almond flour, coconut sugar, melted coconut oil, eggs, vanilla extract, cinnamon, baking powder, baking soda, and salt.
3. Mix until all ingredients are well combined.
4. Pour the batter into the prepared loaf pan and spread it evenly.
5. Bake in the preheated oven for 50-60 minutes, or until a toothpick inserted into the center comes out clean.
6. Let the zucchini bread cool in the pan for 10 minutes, then transfer it to a wire rack to cool completely.
7. Slice and enjoy this moist and flavorful zucchini bread as a healthy dessert or snack option.

4. **Oatmeal Raisin Cookies**
   - o *Ingredients:*

1. 1 cup rolled oats
2. 3/4 cup whole wheat flour
3. 1/2 teaspoon baking soda
4. 1/2 teaspoon ground cinnamon
5. 1/4 teaspoon salt
6. 1/4 cup coconut oil, melted
7. 1/4 cup maple syrup

8. 1/4 cup unsweetened applesauce
9. 1/2 cup raisins

o *Instructions:*

1. Preheat oven to 350°F (175°C). Line a baking sheet with parchment paper.
2. In a large bowl, combine rolled oats, whole wheat flour, baking soda, cinnamon, and salt.
3. In a separate bowl, whisk together melted coconut oil, maple syrup, and unsweetened applesauce.
4. Pour the wet ingredients into the dry ingredients and mix until well combined.
5. Fold in the raisins.
6. Drop spoonfuls of the cookie dough onto the prepared baking sheet.
7. Flatten each cookie with the back of a spoon.
8. Bake in the preheated oven for 10-12 minutes, or until cookies are golden brown.
9. Let cool on the baking sheet for 5 minutes, then transfer to a wire rack to cool completely.
10. Enjoy these wholesome oatmeal raisin cookies as a satisfying dessert or snack.

5. **Avocado Chocolate Mousse**

o *Ingredients:*

1. 2 ripe avocados
2. 1/4 cup cocoa powder
3. 1/4 cup maple syrup or honey
4. 1 teaspoon vanilla extract
5. Pinch of salt

o *Instructions:*

1. Scoop the flesh of the ripe avocados into a food processor.
2. Add cocoa powder, maple syrup or honey, vanilla extract, and a pinch of salt.
3. Blend until smooth and creamy, scraping down the sides of the food processor as needed.
4. Transfer the avocado chocolate mousse to serving dishes.
5. Refrigerate for at least 30 minutes before serving.
6. Garnish with fresh berries or shaved chocolate if desired.
7. Enjoy this rich and indulgent avocado chocolate mousse as a healthier alternative to traditional chocolate desserts.

# Satisfying Sweet Treats

Indulging in sweet treats while managing Parkinson's disease can be both delightful and health-conscious. These recipes focus on using wholesome ingredients to create satisfying desserts that support your nutritional goals.

1. **Berry Chia Jam Bars**
   - **Ingredients:**
     - 1 cup almond flour
     - 1 cup rolled oats
     - 1/2 cup coconut oil, melted
     - 1/4 cup honey or maple syrup
     - 1 cup mixed berries (strawberries, blueberries, raspberries)

- 2 tablespoons chia seeds

- o **Instructions:**

  - Preheat oven to 350°F (175°C) and line a baking dish with parchment paper.
  - In a small saucepan, cook the mixed berries over medium heat until they break down and become syrupy. Stir in chia seeds and let sit for 10 minutes to thicken.
  - In a bowl, combine almond flour, rolled oats, coconut oil, and honey/maple syrup. Mix until a crumbly dough forms.
  - Press half of the dough into the bottom of the baking dish to form a crust.
  - Spread the berry chia jam over the crust.
  - Sprinkle the remaining dough over the top and gently press down.
  - Bake for 20-25 minutes or until the top is golden brown.
  - Let cool before cutting into bars.

2. **Greek Yogurt Parfait**
   - o **Ingredients:**

     - 2 cups Greek yogurt
     - 1/2 cup granola
     - 1 cup mixed berries (blueberries, raspberries, strawberries)
     - 2 tablespoons honey or agave syrup
     - 1 teaspoon vanilla extract

   - o **Instructions:**

     - In a small bowl, mix Greek yogurt with honey/agave syrup and vanilla extract.

- In serving glasses or bowls, layer Greek yogurt, granola, and mixed berries.
- Repeat the layers until the ingredients are used up.
- Serve immediately or refrigerate until ready to eat.

3. **Pumpkin Spice Energy Bites**
   - **Ingredients:**

     - 1 cup rolled oats
     - 1/2 cup pumpkin puree
     - 1/4 cup almond butter
     - 1/4 cup honey or maple syrup
     - 1 teaspoon pumpkin pie spice
     - 1/4 cup dark chocolate chips or dried cranberries

   - **Instructions:**

     - In a large bowl, combine all ingredients and mix well until evenly incorporated.
     - Using your hands, roll the mixture into small balls (about 1 inch in diameter).
     - Place the energy bites on a baking sheet lined with parchment paper.
     - Refrigerate for at least 30 minutes to set.
     - Store in an airtight container in the refrigerator for up to a week.

4. **Mango Coconut Sorbet**
   - **Ingredients:**

     - 3 cups frozen mango chunks
     - 1 cup coconut milk
     - 2 tablespoons honey or agave syrup

- 1 teaspoon lime juice
- o **Instructions:**

  - In a blender or food processor, combine frozen mango, coconut milk, honey/agave syrup, and lime juice.
  - Blend until smooth and creamy.
  - Transfer the mixture to a container and freeze for 2-3 hours until firm.
  - Scoop and serve, garnished with fresh mint or shredded coconut if desired.

5. **Almond Butter Chocolate Cups**
   - o **Ingredients:**

     - 1 cup dark chocolate chips
     - 1/2 cup almond butter
     - 2 tablespoons coconut oil
     - 1 tablespoon honey or maple syrup
     - Sea salt for sprinkling

   - o **Instructions:**

     - Line a muffin tin with paper liners.
     - Melt half of the chocolate chips with 1 tablespoon coconut oil in a microwave-safe bowl in 30-second intervals, stirring until smooth.
     - Divide the melted chocolate among the muffin liners, filling each about 1/4 full. Freeze for 10 minutes to set.
     - In a small bowl, mix almond butter with honey/maple syrup and the remaining coconut oil until smooth.

- Place a spoonful of the almond butter mixture over the set chocolate in each liner.
- Melt the remaining chocolate chips and cover each almond butter layer.
- Sprinkle sea salt on top and freeze for another 10 minutes until firm.
- Store in the refrigerator until ready to serve.

These satisfying sweet treats offer a delightful way to enjoy desserts while supporting a health-conscious diet tailored for Parkinson's disease management. Each recipe is designed to provide nutritional benefits without compromising on flavor and indulgence.

These healthy baking recipes offer delicious ways to satisfy your sweet tooth without compromising on nutrition. Experiment with different ingredients and flavors to customize these treats to your liking.

# PART IV

*LIFESTYLE AND WELLNESS*

## 12. Exercise and Physical Activity

Exercise plays a crucial role in managing Parkinson's disease symptoms and promoting overall well-being. This section explores the benefits of exercise for Parkinson's patients, safe and effective exercise routines, and tips for staying active.

# Benefits of Exercise for Parkinson's Patients

Regular exercise offers numerous benefits for individuals living with Parkinson's disease:

1. **Improved Mobility:** Exercise helps maintain flexibility, balance, and coordination, reducing the risk of falls and improving mobility. Examples include:
     - **Walking:** Taking daily walks outdoors or on a treadmill can enhance cardiovascular health and strengthen leg muscles.
     - **Cycling:** Riding a stationary or outdoor bike can improve leg strength and coordination while providing a low-impact cardiovascular workout.
     - **Dancing:** Participating in dance classes or dancing at home can improve balance, flexibility, and mood while engaging in enjoyable physical activity.
2. **Enhanced Mood:** Physical activity releases endorphins, which can alleviate symptoms of depression and anxiety

commonly associated with Parkinson's disease. Examples include:

- o **Yoga:** Practicing yoga can reduce stress, improve mood, and increase flexibility through gentle stretching and mindful movement.
- o **Tai Chi:** Engaging in tai chi exercises promotes relaxation, mental focus, and balance, contributing to a sense of well-being.

3. **Slowed Disease Progression:** Some studies suggest that exercise may have neuroprotective effects, potentially slowing the progression of Parkinson's disease. Examples include:

- o **Strength Training:** Incorporating resistance exercises using weights, resistance bands, or bodyweight can help maintain muscle strength and slow muscle loss.
- o **High-Intensity Interval Training (HIIT):** Performing short bursts of intense exercise followed by brief rest periods can improve cardiovascular fitness and neuroplasticity.

4. **Increased Strength:** Strength training exercises can help build and maintain muscle strength, making everyday tasks easier to perform. Examples include:

- o **Bodyweight Exercises:** Performing squats, lunges, push-ups, and planks can strengthen major muscle groups without the need for equipment.
- o **Resistance Bands:** Using resistance bands for exercises such as bicep curls, lateral raises, and leg extensions can provide effective strength training workouts at home or in the gym.

5. **Better Quality of Life:** Engaging in regular exercise can enhance overall quality of life by promoting independence, confidence, and a sense of well-being. Examples include:
   - **Group Fitness Classes:** Joining group exercise classes tailored to Parkinson's patients, such as Parkinson's-specific boxing or circuit training, can provide social support and motivation.
   - **Outdoor Activities:** Participating in outdoor recreational activities such as hiking, gardening, or swimming can promote physical fitness while enjoying nature and fresh air.

# Safe and Effective Exercise Routines

When designing an exercise routine for Parkinson's patients, it's essential to focus on activities that address specific symptoms and accommodate individual needs. Here are some safe and effective exercise options:

1. **Cardiovascular Exercise:** Activities such as walking, cycling, swimming, and dancing can improve cardiovascular health, endurance, and stamina.
2. **Strength Training:** Incorporate exercises using resistance bands, free weights, or bodyweight to strengthen muscles and improve functional abilities.
3. **Balance and Flexibility Exercises:** Practices like yoga, tai chi, and Pilates can enhance balance, flexibility, and posture, reducing the risk of falls.
4. **Functional Movement Training:** Focus on exercises that mimic everyday movements, such as reaching, bending, and stepping, to improve functional mobility.

5. **Interval Training:** Alternate between periods of higher intensity and lower intensity exercise to challenge the cardiovascular system and improve overall fitness.

# Tips for Staying Active

Staying motivated and consistent with exercise can be challenging, but incorporating the following tips can help maintain an active lifestyle:

1. **Set Realistic Goals:** Establish achievable exercise goals that align with your abilities and interests, and track your progress to stay motivated.
2. **Find Enjoyable Activities:** Choose exercises that you enjoy and look forward to, whether it's walking in nature, dancing to music, or participating in group fitness classes.
3. **Stay Consistent:** Schedule regular exercise sessions into your weekly routine, and prioritize physical activity as part of your self-care regimen.
4. **Listen to Your Body:** Pay attention to how your body responds to exercise and adjust the intensity or duration as needed to prevent overexertion or injury.
5. **Seek Support:** Enlist the support of friends, family members, or a certified fitness professional who can provide encouragement, accountability, and guidance on safe exercise practices.

By incorporating regular exercise into your routine and adopting a holistic approach to wellness, you can enhance your physical and mental well-being while managing the symptoms of Parkinson's disease effectively.

## 13. Stress Management and Mental Health

Managing stress and prioritizing mental health are essential components of overall well-being, especially for individuals living with Parkinson's disease. This section explores various techniques for reducing stress, mindfulness and meditation practices, and ways to support mental health.

# Techniques for Reducing Stress

Living with Parkinson's disease can be challenging, and stress management techniques can help alleviate symptoms and improve quality of life. Here are some effective strategies for reducing stress:

1. **Deep Breathing Exercises:** Practice deep breathing techniques to calm the nervous system and reduce stress levels. Inhale deeply through your nose, hold for a few seconds, and exhale slowly through your mouth.
2. **Progressive Muscle Relaxation:** Tense and relax different muscle groups in your body to release tension and promote relaxation. Start with your toes and work your way up to your head, focusing on each muscle group individually.
3. **Mindful Movement:** Engage in gentle exercises such as yoga, tai chi, or qigong that incorporate mindful movement and breath awareness. These practices can help reduce stress while improving flexibility, balance, and mental clarity.
4. **Nature Therapy:** Spend time outdoors in nature, whether it's taking a walk in the park, gardening, or simply sitting in a natural setting. Connecting with nature can have a calming effect on the mind and reduce stress levels.
5. **Journaling:** Keep a journal to express your thoughts, feelings, and experiences. Writing can be a therapeutic outlet

for processing emotions and gaining perspective on challenging situations.

6. **Social Support:** Seek support from friends, family members, support groups, or mental health professionals. Sharing your experiences and feelings with others who understand can provide comfort and validation.

# Mindfulness and Meditation Practices

Mindfulness and meditation practices are powerful tools for reducing stress, enhancing self-awareness, and promoting mental well-being. Here are some mindfulness techniques to try:

1. **Body Scan Meditation:** Lie down in a comfortable position and focus your attention on each part of your body, starting from your toes and moving up to your head. Notice any sensations, tensions, or areas of discomfort, and allow them to soften and release with each breath.
2. **Mindful Walking:** Take a slow, deliberate walk while paying attention to each step, the sensation of your feet touching the ground, and the movement of your body. Notice the sights, sounds, and smells around you without judgment.
3. **Breath Awareness:** Sit comfortably and bring your attention to your breath. Notice the natural rhythm of your breathing, the rise and fall of your chest or abdomen, and the sensation of air flowing in and out of your nostrils. Whenever your mind wanders, gently bring your focus back to your breath.
4. **Loving-Kindness Meditation:** Cultivate feelings of compassion and kindness towards yourself and others by silently repeating phrases such as "May I be happy, may I be healthy, may I be at peace." Extend these wishes to loved ones, acquaintances, and all beings.

111

5. **Guided Imagery:** Close your eyes and imagine yourself in a peaceful and serene setting, such as a beach, forest, or mountaintop. Engage all your senses to vividly picture the scene, allowing yourself to relax and let go of tension.

## Supporting Mental Health

Prioritizing mental health is essential for individuals living with Parkinson's disease. Here are some ways to support mental well-being:

1. **Maintain a Healthy Lifestyle:** Eat a balanced diet, engage in regular physical activity, get adequate sleep, and avoid excessive alcohol consumption and smoking. These lifestyle factors can impact mood, energy levels, and overall mental health.
2. **Stay Connected:** Maintain social connections with friends, family members, and support groups. Share your experiences, concerns, and triumphs with others who understand and offer encouragement.
3. **Seek Professional Support:** If you're struggling with stress, anxiety, depression, or other mental health challenges, don't hesitate to seek help from a qualified mental health professional. Therapy, counseling, and medication can be valuable resources for managing symptoms and improving well-being.
4. **Practice Self-Compassion:** Be kind and compassionate towards yourself, especially during difficult times. Treat yourself with the same understanding and empathy that you would offer to a friend facing similar challenges.
5. **Engage in Activities You Enjoy:** Make time for hobbies, interests, and activities that bring you joy and fulfillment.

Whether it's reading, painting, listening to music, or spending time in nature, engaging in pleasurable activities can boost mood and reduce stress.

By incorporating stress management techniques, mindfulness practices, and strategies for supporting mental health into your daily routine, you can cultivate resilience, enhance coping skills, and improve your overall quality of life while living with Parkinson's disease.

## 14. Sleep and Rest

Ensuring adequate sleep and rest is crucial for maintaining overall health and well-being, especially for individuals living with Parkinson's disease. This section highlights the importance of sleep for brain health, provides tips for improving sleep quality, and discusses creating a restful sleep environment.

# Importance of Sleep for Brain Health

Quality sleep is essential for various cognitive functions, emotional well-being, and overall brain health. For individuals with Parkinson's disease, adequate sleep plays a critical role in managing symptoms and optimizing daily functioning. Here are some key reasons why sleep is important for brain health:

1. **Memory Consolidation:** During sleep, the brain processes and consolidates information gathered throughout the day, enhancing learning and memory retention.

2. **Brain Restoration:** Sleep allows the brain to repair and regenerate cells, promoting neural growth and plasticity, which are essential for cognitive function and mental clarity.
3. **Emotional Regulation:** Adequate sleep is essential for regulating emotions and mood stability. Sleep deprivation can lead to increased irritability, anxiety, and depressive symptoms.
4. **Motor Function:** Quality sleep supports optimal motor function and coordination, which can help mitigate symptoms such as tremors, stiffness, and bradykinesia associated with Parkinson's disease.
5. **Immune Function:** Sleep plays a vital role in regulating the immune system, promoting immune response and defense against infections and inflammation, which can impact overall health and disease progression.

## Tips for Improving Sleep Quality

Improving sleep quality is essential for individuals with Parkinson's disease to manage symptoms effectively and enhance overall well-being. Here are some tips for achieving better sleep:

1. **Establish a Consistent Sleep Schedule:** Go to bed and wake up at the same time each day, even on weekends, to regulate your body's internal clock and promote healthy sleep-wake cycles.
2. **Create a Relaxing Bedtime Routine:** Develop a calming bedtime routine to signal to your body that it's time to wind down. Activities such as reading, gentle stretching, listening to soothing music, or taking a warm bath can help promote relaxation and prepare you for sleep.

3. **Limit Screen Time Before Bed:** Avoid electronic devices such as smartphones, tablets, and computers at least an hour before bedtime, as the blue light emitted from screens can disrupt melatonin production and interfere with sleep quality.

4. **Optimize Sleep Environment:** Make your bedroom conducive to sleep by keeping it dark, quiet, and cool. Use blackout curtains, white noise machines, or earplugs to block out any disruptive noises or light sources.

5. **Limit Stimulants and Alcohol:** Avoid consuming caffeine and alcohol close to bedtime, as they can interfere with sleep quality and disrupt sleep cycles.

6. **Manage Symptoms:** Address any symptoms of Parkinson's disease that may disrupt sleep, such as tremors, stiffness, or urinary urgency. Work with your healthcare provider to develop a management plan that minimizes symptom impact on sleep.

# Creating a Restful Sleep Environment

Creating a restful sleep environment is essential for promoting quality sleep and optimizing restorative rest. Here are some strategies for creating an ideal sleep environment:

1. **Invest in a Comfortable Mattress and Bedding:** Choose a mattress and bedding that provide adequate support and comfort to promote restful sleep. Consider factors such as mattress firmness, pillow support, and breathable fabrics to create a cozy sleep environment.

2. **Minimize Light Exposure:** Use blackout curtains or shades to block out external light sources that can disrupt sleep. Consider using a sleep mask if you're unable to eliminate all light sources in your bedroom.

3. **Reduce Noise Disturbances:** Use earplugs or a white noise machine to block out disruptive noises such as traffic, snoring, or household sounds that may interfere with sleep.

4. **Maintain Comfortable Temperature:** Keep your bedroom cool and comfortable, as temperature can impact sleep quality. Experiment with room temperature settings and bedding options to find the optimal sleep environment for you.

5. **Declutter Your Bedroom:** Keep your bedroom free of clutter and distractions to promote relaxation and calmness. Remove electronic devices, work-related materials, and other stimuli that may cause stress or anxiety before bedtime.

By prioritizing sleep and implementing strategies for improving sleep quality and creating a restful sleep environment, individuals with Parkinson's disease can enhance their overall health, well-being, and quality of life. It's essential to work with healthcare providers to address any underlying sleep disorders or symptoms that may impact sleep quality and to tailor strategies to individual needs and preferences.

## 15. Social Support and Community

Building a strong support network and fostering connections within the Parkinson's community can provide invaluable resources, guidance, and emotional support for individuals living with Parkinson's disease and their caregivers. This section emphasizes the importance of social support, highlights resources available for Parkinson's patients and caregivers, and explores the benefits of joining support groups and communities.

# Building a Support Network

Navigating life with Parkinson's disease can be challenging, but having a supportive network of friends, family, healthcare professionals, and fellow patients can make a significant difference. Here are some strategies for building a support network:

1. **Communicate Openly:** Share your experiences, concerns, and needs with trusted individuals in your life. Open communication fosters understanding and strengthens relationships.
2. **Educate Your Loved Ones:** Help your friends and family members understand Parkinson's disease by providing educational materials, attending medical appointments together, and engaging in honest conversations about your condition.
3. **Seek Professional Support:** Consult with healthcare providers, including neurologists, physical therapists, occupational therapists, and mental health professionals, who can offer guidance, treatment options, and specialized care tailored to your needs.
4. **Connect with Other Patients:** Reach out to other individuals living with Parkinson's disease through local support groups, online forums, and community events. Sharing experiences and tips with others who understand can provide validation, encouragement, and practical advice.
5. **Involve Caregivers:** If you have caregivers or family members supporting you, involve them in your care plan and provide opportunities for them to access resources, respite care, and support services to prevent burnout and promote their well-being.

# Resources for Parkinson's Patients and Caregivers

Numerous resources are available to support individuals living with Parkinson's disease and their caregivers. These resources offer information, education, advocacy, and practical assistance. Some key resources include:

1. **Parkinson's Disease Foundation (PDF):** PDF offers a wide range of educational materials, webinars, support groups, and resources for patients, caregivers, and healthcare professionals.
2. **Michael J. Fox Foundation for Parkinson's Research:** The Michael J. Fox Foundation funds research, provides educational resources, and advocates for policies that benefit Parkinson's patients and their families.
3. **National Parkinson Foundation (NPF):** NPF offers educational programs, support groups, and community events for Parkinson's patients and caregivers, as well as resources for healthcare professionals.
4. **Davis Phinney Foundation:** The Davis Phinney Foundation provides resources, tools, and programs focused on living well with Parkinson's disease, including educational materials, exercise programs, and community events.
5. **Local Support Groups:** Many communities have local Parkinson's support groups that offer meetings, educational sessions, and social events for patients and caregivers. Contact your local hospital, Parkinson's clinic, or advocacy organization to find support groups in your area.

# Joining Support Groups and Communities

Joining support groups and communities can provide a sense of belonging, validation, and empowerment for individuals living with Parkinson's disease and their caregivers. Benefits of participating in support groups include:

1. **Shared Understanding:** Connecting with others who share similar experiences can provide validation, empathy, and understanding, reducing feelings of isolation and loneliness.
2. **Practical Advice:** Support groups offer opportunities to exchange tips, strategies, and resources for managing symptoms, navigating healthcare systems, and accessing community services.
3. **Emotional Support:** Sharing concerns, fears, and triumphs in a supportive environment can alleviate stress, anxiety, and depression, promoting emotional well-being and resilience.
4. **Education and Empowerment:** Support groups often feature educational presentations, guest speakers, and workshops on topics relevant to Parkinson's disease, empowering participants with knowledge and advocacy skills.
5. **Social Connection:** Participating in support groups fosters social connections and friendships, providing opportunities for companionship, recreation, and mutual support outside of formal meetings.

By actively building a support network, accessing available resources, and engaging with support groups and communities, individuals living with Parkinson's disease and their caregivers can enhance their quality of life, improve coping skills, and navigate the challenges of Parkinson's disease with resilience and hope.

# PART V



## 16. Supplements and Alternative Therapies

Exploring supplements and alternative therapies can be a complementary approach to managing Parkinson's disease symptoms and promoting overall well-being. This section provides an overview of common supplements, guidance for evaluating alternative therapies, and the importance of consulting with healthcare providers.

## Overview of Common Supplements

While research on the effectiveness of supplements for Parkinson's disease is ongoing, some individuals find certain supplements beneficial in managing symptoms or supporting overall health. Common supplements used by individuals with Parkinson's disease include:

1. **Coenzyme Q10 (CoQ10):** CoQ10 is an antioxidant that plays a role in cellular energy production. Some studies suggest that CoQ10 supplementation may have neuroprotective effects and improve motor symptoms in Parkinson's patients.
2. **Vitamin B6 (Pyridoxine):** Vitamin B6 is involved in neurotransmitter synthesis and may help alleviate symptoms such as depression and fatigue in Parkinson's patients. However, excessive intake of vitamin B6 can cause neuropathy, so it's essential to monitor dosage.

3. **Vitamin D:** Vitamin D deficiency is common in individuals with Parkinson's disease and may contribute to bone health issues and cognitive impairment. Supplementing with vitamin D may help maintain bone density and support overall health.

4. **Omega-3 Fatty Acids:** Omega-3 fatty acids, found in fish oil supplements, have anti-inflammatory properties and may support brain health and cognitive function. Some studies suggest that omega-3 supplementation may help reduce inflammation and oxidative stress in Parkinson's patients.

5. **N-Acetylcysteine (NAC):** NAC is an antioxidant that may help protect against oxidative damage and inflammation in the brain. Preliminary research suggests that NAC supplementation may improve motor symptoms and cognitive function in Parkinson's disease.

6. **Green Tea Extract:** Green tea contains polyphenols such as epigallocatechin gallate (EGCG), which have antioxidant and neuroprotective properties. Some studies suggest that green tea extract supplementation may help alleviate oxidative stress and improve motor function in Parkinson's patients.

It's important to note that supplements should not replace conventional Parkinson's disease treatments prescribed by healthcare providers. Before starting any supplements, individuals should consult with their healthcare team to ensure safety and effectiveness, as well as to avoid potential interactions with medications.

## Evaluating Alternative Therapies

In addition to supplements, individuals with Parkinson's disease may explore alternative therapies to manage symptoms and improve quality of life. Some alternative therapies commonly used by Parkinson's patients include:

1. **Acupuncture:** Acupuncture involves the insertion of thin needles into specific points on the body to promote balance and alleviate symptoms. Some individuals find acupuncture helpful for reducing pain, stiffness, and tremors associated with Parkinson's disease.
2. **Massage Therapy:** Massage therapy can help alleviate muscle stiffness, tension, and pain, improving mobility and relaxation. Gentle massage techniques tailored to individual needs may provide relief from Parkinson's symptoms.
3. **Tai Chi and Qigong:** Tai Chi and Qigong are mind-body practices that involve slow, deliberate movements, breathing exercises, and meditation. These practices promote balance, flexibility, and relaxation, which can benefit individuals with Parkinson's disease.
4. **Music Therapy:** Music therapy involves listening to or creating music to promote emotional expression, communication, and relaxation. Some studies suggest that music therapy may improve mood, cognitive function, and motor skills in Parkinson's patients.
5. **Dance Therapy:** Dance therapy combines movement and music to improve physical, emotional, and cognitive well-being. Dancing can enhance balance, coordination, and mood while providing a creative outlet for self-expression.

Before trying any alternative therapies, individuals should discuss their options with their healthcare providers to ensure safety and appropriateness, especially if they have underlying health conditions or are taking medications that may interact with certain therapies.

# Consulting with Healthcare Providers

While supplements and alternative therapies may offer potential benefits for managing Parkinson's disease symptoms, it's essential to approach them with caution and consult with healthcare providers before making any changes to treatment plans. Healthcare providers can offer guidance, monitor for potential interactions or adverse effects, and help individuals make informed decisions about incorporating supplements and alternative therapies into their care.

Individuals with Parkinson's disease should maintain open communication with their healthcare team and inform them of any supplements or alternative therapies they are considering. Healthcare providers can provide personalized recommendations based on individual needs, preferences, and treatment goals, ensuring safe and effective integration of supplements and alternative therapies into comprehensive Parkinson's disease management plans.

## 17. FAQs and Troubleshooting

This section addresses common questions about the Parkinson's diet, provides guidance for troubleshooting dietary challenges, and offers tips for adjusting the diet to meet individual needs.

# Common Questions About the Parkinson's Diet

1.  **What foods should I include in a Parkinson's diet?**
    o   A Parkinson's diet should prioritize nutrient-dense foods such as fruits, vegetables, whole grains, lean proteins, and healthy fats. Incorporating foods rich in

antioxidants, vitamins, and minerals can help support brain health and overall well-being.

2. **Are there any foods I should avoid with Parkinson's disease?**
   - While there is no specific diet for Parkinson's disease, some individuals may find that certain foods or dietary habits worsen their symptoms. Common triggers include highly processed foods, excess sugar, caffeine, and alcohol. It's essential to pay attention to how your body responds to different foods and adjust your diet accordingly.

3. **Should I follow a specific meal timing or eating schedule?**
   - While there is no one-size-fits-all approach to meal timing, some individuals with Parkinson's disease may benefit from eating smaller, more frequent meals throughout the day to maintain energy levels and manage medication absorption. Experiment with different eating schedules to find what works best for you.

4. **Is there a role for supplements in managing Parkinson's symptoms?**
   - Some individuals with Parkinson's disease may benefit from certain supplements to address nutritional deficiencies or support overall health. However, it's essential to consult with a healthcare provider before starting any supplements, as they may interact with medications or have adverse effects.

5. **How can I maintain a healthy weight with Parkinson's disease?**
   - Eating a balanced diet rich in nutrient-dense foods and engaging in regular physical activity can help support weight management and overall health. If you're

experiencing unintended weight loss or gain, consult with a healthcare provider or registered dietitian for personalized guidance and support.

**Troubleshooting Dietary Challenges**

1. **Difficulty Swallowing (Dysphagia):**
   - If swallowing becomes challenging due to Parkinson's symptoms, focus on softer, easier-to-swallow foods such as smoothies, soups, pureed vegetables, and yogurt. Consult with a speech therapist or registered dietitian for guidance on modifying textures and maintaining adequate nutrition.
2. **Loss of Appetite:**
   - If Parkinson's symptoms or medication side effects contribute to a loss of appetite, try eating smaller, more frequent meals throughout the day and incorporating nutrient-dense snacks between meals. Focus on calorie-rich foods such as nuts, nut butter, avocado, and dairy products to boost energy intake.
3. **Gastrointestinal Symptoms (Constipation, Nausea, Bloating):**
   - To alleviate gastrointestinal symptoms, prioritize fiber-rich foods such as fruits, vegetables, whole grains, and legumes to support digestive health and regularity. Stay hydrated by drinking plenty of water throughout the day, and consider incorporating probiotic-rich foods such as yogurt, kefir, and fermented vegetables to promote gut health.
4. **Medication Interactions:**
   - Be mindful of potential interactions between Parkinson's medications and certain foods or dietary supplements. Some medications may require specific

timing in relation to meals or interactions with certain nutrients. Consult with a healthcare provider or pharmacist for guidance on medication management and dietary considerations.

# Adjusting the Diet for Individual Needs

1. **Personal Preferences:**
   - Tailor your Parkinson's diet to accommodate personal preferences, cultural traditions, and dietary restrictions. Experiment with different recipes, cooking methods, and flavor profiles to make healthy eating enjoyable and sustainable.
2. **Nutritional Needs:**
   - Consider your individual nutritional needs based on factors such as age, gender, activity level, and medical history. Work with a registered dietitian to develop a personalized nutrition plan that meets your specific dietary requirements and health goals.
3. **Symptom Management:**
   - Adjust your diet to address specific Parkinson's symptoms or medication side effects. For example, if you experience constipation, focus on fiber-rich foods and adequate hydration. If you have difficulty swallowing, choose softer textures and smaller, more frequent meals.
4. **Long-Term Sustainability:**
   - Aim for a balanced, flexible approach to eating that promotes long-term health and well-being. Incorporate a variety of foods from all food groups, and practice mindful eating to cultivate a positive

relationship with food and nourish your body effectively.

By addressing common questions, troubleshooting dietary challenges, and adjusting the diet to meet individual needs, individuals with Parkinson's disease can optimize nutrition, manage symptoms effectively, and enhance overall quality of life. It's essential to consult with healthcare providers and registered dietitians for personalized guidance and support in navigating dietary considerations related to Parkinson's disease.

## 18. Appendices

# Glossary of Terms

- **Bradykinesia:** Slowness of movement, a common symptom of Parkinson's disease characterized by a gradual loss of spontaneous movement and a general reduction in the speed of voluntary movements.
- **Dyskinesia:** Involuntary, erratic, and uncontrollable movements that can occur as a side effect of Parkinson's medications, particularly levodopa.
- **Freezing of Gait (FOG):** A sudden, temporary inability to move the feet forward while walking, often described as feeling "stuck" to the ground, which can occur in Parkinson's disease.
- **Levodopa:** A medication commonly used to treat Parkinson's disease, which is converted into dopamine in the brain to replenish dopamine levels and alleviate motor symptoms.
- **Neurotransmitter:** Chemical messengers in the brain that transmit signals between nerve cells, including dopamine, which is deficient in Parkinson's disease.

- **Tremor:** Involuntary shaking or trembling of a limb or body part, often seen as a characteristic symptom of Parkinson's disease.

# Measurement Conversions

- 1 cup = 240 milliliters
- 1 tablespoon = 15 milliliters
- 1 teaspoon = 5 milliliters
- 1 ounce = 28 grams
- 1 pound = 454 grams
- 1 inch = 2.54 centimeters
- 1 kilogram = 2.2 pounds
- 1 liter = 1,000 milliliters

# Index of Recipes

- **Breakfast:**
    - Nutritious Breakfast Smoothies
    - High-Protein Breakfast Options
    - Easy-to-Prepare Breakfast Ideas
- **Lunch:**
    - Brain-Boosting Salads
    - Hearty Soups and Stews
    - Simple Sandwiches and Wraps
- **Dinner:**
    - Balanced Main Courses
    - Vegetarian and Vegan Options
    - Slow Cooker Recipes for Convenience
- **Snacks and Sides:**
    - Healthy Snack Ideas
    - Nutritious Side Dishes

- o Quick Bites for Energy
- **Desserts and Treats:**
  - o Low-Sugar Dessert Options
  - o Healthy Baking Recipes
  - o Satisfying Sweet Treats

By providing a glossary of terms, measurement conversions, and an index of recipes, the appendices serve as valuable reference materials for readers of the Parkinson's disease diet cookbook. These resources enhance understanding, facilitate meal preparation, and promote accessibility to the content presented in the book.

# Conclusion

## 19. Final Thoughts

As we conclude this comprehensive journey through the Parkinson's disease diet cookbook, it's essential to reflect on the wealth of knowledge acquired, the practical strategies explored, and the profound impact these insights can have on your health and well-being.

## Reflecting on Your Journey

Throughout this insightful exploration, you've delved deep into the intricate relationship between nutrition and Parkinson's disease management. From understanding the role of nutrient-rich foods in supporting brain health to discovering practical meal planning and preparation techniques, you've equipped yourself with invaluable tools for optimizing your dietary habits and enhancing your quality of life.

Take a moment to reflect on how this newfound knowledge has transformed your approach to nutrition and empowered you to take proactive steps towards better health. Celebrate the progress you've made and the positive changes you've implemented along the way.

## Staying Motivated and Informed

As you continue your journey with Parkinson's disease, it's crucial to remain motivated, informed, and engaged in your health and well-being. Stay connected with a network of healthcare providers, support groups, and resources within the Parkinson's community to access ongoing education, support, and guidance.

Keep abreast of the latest research findings, emerging therapies, and innovative approaches to Parkinson's disease management. By staying informed and proactive, you can navigate the complexities of Parkinson's disease with confidence and resilience.

## Looking Forward

As you embark on the next chapter of your journey, embrace the future with optimism, determination, and a steadfast commitment to your health. Continue to prioritize self-care, nourish your body with wholesome foods, and cultivate a positive mindset that fosters resilience and well-being.

Embrace the journey ahead as an opportunity for growth, exploration, and personal empowerment. Remember that every step you take towards optimizing your nutrition and lifestyle is a step towards enhancing your vitality, resilience, and overall quality of life.

In closing, may this cookbook serve as a cherished companion on your path to wellness, providing inspiration, guidance, and nourishment for both body and soul. As you navigate the road ahead, may you find joy, fulfillment, and abundant health in every moment.

With warmest regards,

Dr. Sarah Matthews

# References

<u>20. Citations and Further Reading</u>


1. Ascherio, A., & Schwarzschild, M. A. (2016). The epidemiology of Parkinson's disease: risk factors and prevention. The Lancet Neurology, 15(12), 1257-1272.
2. Cereda, E., Barichella, M., Cassani, E., Caccialanza, R., Pezzoli, G., & Tesei, S. (2017). Dietary habits and neurological features of Parkinson's disease patients: implications for practice. Clinical Nutrition, 36(4), 1054-1061.
3. Fereshtehnejad, S. M., Ghazi, L., Shafieesabet, M., Shahidi, G. A., & Delbari, A. (2015). Locus coeruleus degeneration and Parkinson's disease: a clinical-pathologic study. Acta Neuropathologica Communications, 3(1), 1-8.
4. Mischley, L. K., Lau, R. C., & Bennett, R. D. (2017). Role of diet and nutritional supplements in Parkinson's disease progression. Oxidative Medicine and Cellular Longevity, 2017.
5. National Parkinson Foundation. (n.d.). Diet and Parkinson's Disease. Retrieved from https://www.parkinson.org/Living-with-Parkinsons/Managing-Parkinsons/Diet-and-Nutrition.

# Recommended Books and Websites

1. "The Parkinson's Playbook: A Game Plan to Put Your Parkinson's Disease on the Defense" by Robert Smith
2. "Goodbye Parkinson's, Hello Life!: The Gyro–Kinetic Method for Eliminating Symptoms and Reclaiming Your Good Health" by Alex Kerten
3. "Parkinson's Foundation" - https://www.parkinson.org/
4. "Michael J. Fox Foundation for Parkinson's Research" - https://www.michaeljfox.org/
5. "Davis Phinney Foundation" - https://davisphinneyfoundation.org/

## Contact Information for Parkinson's Organizations

1. Parkinson's Foundation
   - Phone: 1-800-4PD-INFO (1-800-473-4636)
   - Email: helpline@parkinson.org
   - Website: https://www.parkinson.org/
2. Michael J. Fox Foundation for Parkinson's Research
   - Phone: 1-800-708-7644
   - Email: info@michaeljfox.org
   - Website: https://www.michaeljfox.org/
3. Davis Phinney Foundation
   - Phone: 1-866-358-0285
   - Email: contact@dpf.org
   - Website: https://davisphinneyfoundation.org/

These organizations offer a wealth of resources, support services, and educational materials for individuals living with Parkinson's disease and their caregivers. Don't hesitate to reach out for assistance, information, or to get involved in research and advocacy efforts.

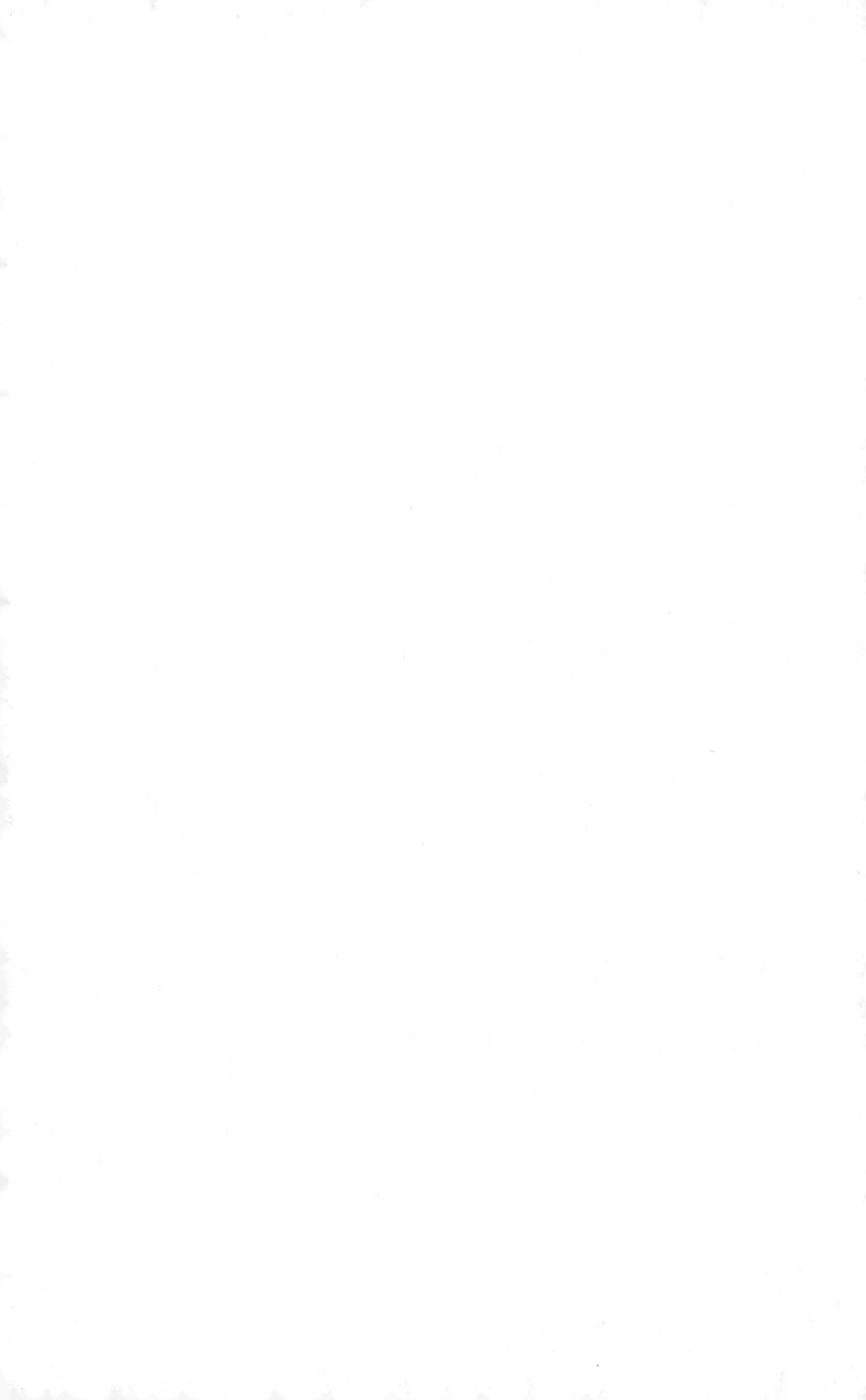